ISBN 978-1-899845-19-4

Glasgow Veterinary School 1862-2012

Glasgow Vets 1862–2012

150

Celebrating 150 years of veterinary excellence

Creators

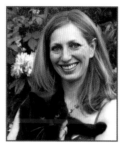

Editor-in-Chief
Dr Philippa Yam

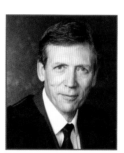

Editors
Professor Peter Holmes

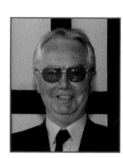

Professor Max Murray

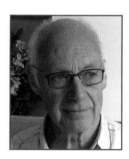

Professor Os Jarrettt

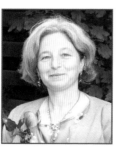

Research Assistant
Ms Julie Kennedy

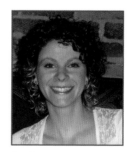

Graphic Designer
Ms Jenna Pollock

Acknowledgments

Writing a book about the 150 years since the founding of Glasgow Veterinary School in 1862 has been a huge undertaking and could not possibly have been completed without the many contributions of recollections, pictures and historical facts from members of staff, alumni, students and friends of the School. We are extremely grateful to you all. Every effort has been made to give an accurate account of the School's history and any omissions or inaccuracies are regretted.

I would like to thank a few people in particular for their support in the researching, writing and help with the editing of this book. Julie Kennedy, Research Assistant, has an amazing capacity for sourcing both information and images, especially from those early days in James McCall's era, and has worked ceaselessly over the last year collating images, writing and referencing this book. Many thanks to Peter Holmes, Max Murray and Os Jarrett who have been integral to the writing of this book and Max in particular, has provided images gathered over many years; between them they have a wealth of information about the development of our School.

Images have come from a variety of other sources including, archive images, with permission of University of Glasgow Archive Services and help from Lesley Richmond, Moira Rankin, Alma Topen, duty archivists, assistants and trainees of University of Glasgow Archives Services. The team were very helpful in suggesting, finding, photographing and scanning images.

Also we would like to thank Tim Amyes, Secretary Scottish Motor Museum Trust; South Lanarkshire Council; Geraldine McCall for providing McCall family photographs and information; SCRAN/ RCAHMS Enterprises for the Veterinary Surgery, Rutherglen; Medical Illustration, Glasgow Royal Infirmary for the Lister photograph; the University of Glasgow Library for providing maps of Sauchiehall Lane and Buccleuch Street; staff of University of Glasgow Special Collections for George Armatage plates; and the University of Glasgow Photography Unit. Every effort has been made to trace and acknowledge copyright.

A number of individuals have assisted in research and include Lesley Richmond and staff of University of Glasgow Archives Services; Carol Parry of the Royal College of Physicians and Surgeons of Glasgow; Caroline Hutchinson, Operations Manager, who has a wealth of knowledge about staff and students; Jimmy Armour; Maureen McGovern and Craig Brennan, Vet School Librarians; Sarah Hunter in the Development and Alumni Office; Alison McClary, Library Assistant, RCVS Charitable Trust; Colin Warwick and Alasdair MacDonald, Royal (Dick) School of Veterinary Studies, and Willie Johnston, University of Edinburgh.

I would like to express thanks for financial assistance from the Chancellors Fund, University of Glasgow, the Carnegie Trust of the Universities of Scotland and the Guthrie Trust, Scottish Society of the History of Medicine.

Finally, I express my gratitude to Jenna Pollock, graphic designer 'extraordinaire' for her invaluable expertise and patience.

Philippa Yam, 2012

Foreword

It is a great privilege to have been asked to write the foreword to this book, which celebrates 150 years of veterinary study and research in Glasgow.

As I struggle to find words worthy to preface our history I am sitting on an aeroplane gazing down at the River Danube, disappearing into the distant haze as it winds its way through the central plain of Europe. Like many wonderful things in nature it leaves me feeling humbled and diminished. The sheer scale of it, and the volume of water flowing every minute, one can only imagine all the things it has passed over the centuries. The river as a metaphor for a journey through time is hardly original but does seem particularly apt when contemplating the school and its history of learning and enquiry; a body of knowledge that inexorably swells with the passage of time. How all the little tributaries contribute to the stream of learning, and how ideas and discoveries have irrigated the lands far beyond the banks of the river illustrates our journey over the last 150 years.

Within the pages of this book you will find the names of men and women who have advanced our understanding of animal diseases, carefully exploring and recording the intricate and perpetual dance between pathogens and their hosts. Also described are pioneers who have mapped the complex changes that corrupt health and developed strategies and treatments to improve the lot of animals. However, I want to pay tribute not only to the big names and famous discoveries recorded here but to all those that have contributed to our enlightenment over the last fifteen decades, too many to be mentioned in the pages that follow. The real beauty of enquiry is that it is a journey to an unknown destination with many carrying the baton for a brief period.

Higher education is a place to ponder and debate new ideas, a place to advance thinking and stimulate fresh minds. In this tradition we can be proud of our history at Glasgow and be hopeful for the future. The impact of our teaching and the passing of accumulated knowledge from one generation to the next cannot be underestimated.

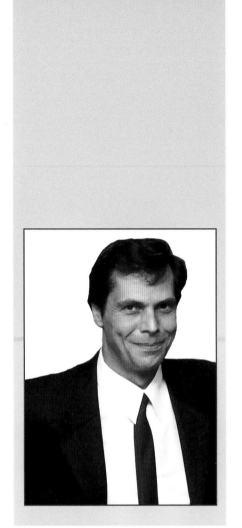

Ewan Cameron

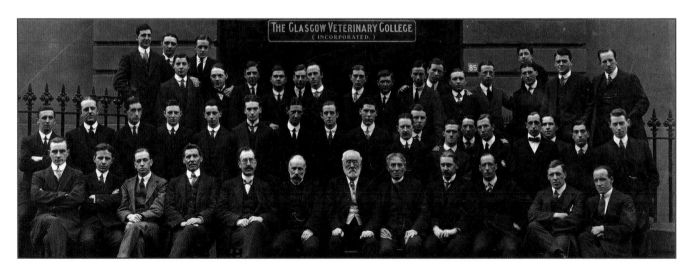

Staff and students of the Glasgow Veterinary College 1913-1914

I am struck by the force for good that one Vet School can achieve; graduates between 1862 and 2012 who have gone across the world tackling disease and suffering at the national level, the herd level and in the individual animal.

Veterinary medicine has come a long way in the last century and a half but some things do not change; the desire to ensure the welfare of animals and the determination to support the farmer, the herder and the individual owner through the good times and the bad. We are vets who care deeply about our calling and our responsibilities and who cherish the importance of stock and companion animals to society. This is an opportunity to praise the work of the practioner, 150 years worth of treating animals day in and day out, 150 years of making the world a better place. The progress since 1862 has been driven by the desire to know more, to understand better, to embrace the discipline and rigour of science and apply it to practice. This is indeed a heritage to be proud of. The Danube is disappearing into the far yonder but it is going to be exciting to find out what is around the next bend of the river. It has been an adventurous journey so far and the future looks promising!

Ewan Cameron, May 2012

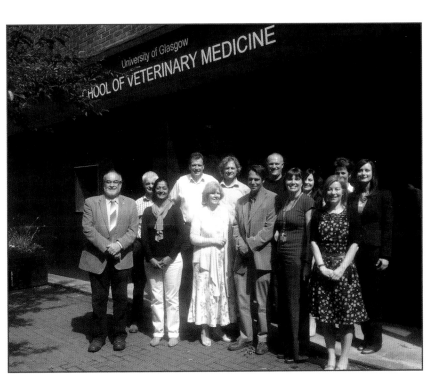

School Executive 2012

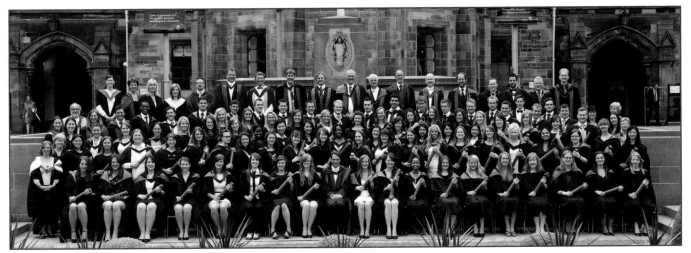

Glasgow Vet School graduation 2012

Chapter 1:
The McCall Years 1862-1915

The beginning   08
James McCall: founder and   09
first Principal
Early days   10
Move to Buccleuch Street   12
Glasgow Veterinary College   14
incorporated as a public institution
McCall family history   15

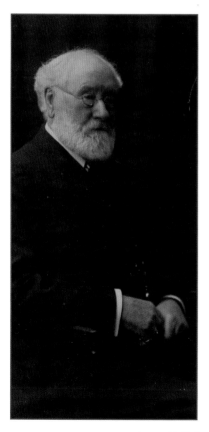

James McCall

Chapter 2:
The Pre-University College 1915-1949

New era, new Principals   18
Principal Hugh Begg 1915-1917   19
Principal Sidney Gaiger 1917-1922   19
Early research in Buccleuch Street   19
Principal Arthur Whitehouse 1922-1945   19
The Constable Report   20
The Loveday Committee   21
First Scottish women veterinary   21
students
Alf Wight 1939 graduate   23
Eddie Straiton 1940 graduate   23
The Loveday Report revisited 1944   24
The last Principals of the old College   24
Donald Campbell (1945-1946) and
Albert Forsyth (1946-1949)
Student memories of Buccleuch Street   25
in the 1940s

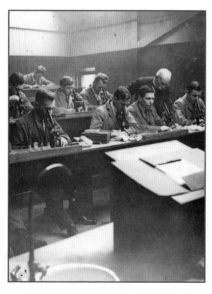

*Physiology Laboratory, Dr John Lindsay
demonstrating to students c1930*

Chapter 3:
Veterinary Education in the University Era

New Director, William Weipers   28
Student days: work hard play hard   31
Staff, old and new   32
George Barr 1955 graduate   33
Student admissions   33
New curriculum   33
Practical experience off-site   35
Sporting vets   35
Jimmy Murphy   35
Undergraduate research training   36
Freshers social and the Garscube   36
Gazette
Vet School Centenary 1962   37
The Faculty of Veterinary Medicine   37
Ian McIntyre Dean 1974-1977   37
New professors - real and titular   37
Bill Mulligan Dean 1977-1980   38
Purchase of the Lanark Practice   38
A lecture-free final year   38
Donald Lawson Dean 1980-1983   39
The Riley Report   40
Tom Douglas Dean 1983-1986   40
Jimmy Armour Dean 1986-1991   40
Glasgow moves forward   41
Norman Wright Dean 1991-1999   41
Curriculum continues to evolve   41
Clinical Scholars Programme   41
Andrea Nolan Dean 1999-2004   42
Fifty & Forwards 1949 - 1999   42
Veterinary Nursing   43
Overseas Veterinary Students and   43
Accreditation
Student numbers and gender balance   45
Modern teaching innovations towards   45
the 21st century
New century and new courses   47
The BVMS programme: into the future   48
Stuart Reid Dean 2005-2010   49
Ewan Cameron, Head of School 2011   49

Chapter 4:
Discovery and Innovation

Weipers' vision of 'One Medicine'   52
Parasitology   53
Ruminant helminths   53
Bovine lungworm   54
Bovine parasitic gastritis   55
Liver fluke disease   56
Other gastric nematodes   56
Equine helminths   57
Mechanisms of immunity to parasites   57
Pathophysiology of parasitic infections   58
Pharmacokinetics of anti-parasite drugs   59
Molecular biology of parasites   59
Genetic resistance to helminth infections   61
Virology   62
Canine virology   63
Feline virology   65
Molecular oncology   68
The Leukaemia Research Fund Virus Centre   68
Bovine viral diseases   69
Equine sarcoid   70
Bacteriology   71
Neuroscience   73
The Wellcome Surgical Institute   73
Neurology   74
Orthopaedic research   75
Animal health and production   77
Cattle diseases   77
Ruminant nutrition   78
Reproductive physiology   79
Aquaculture   80
Poultry research   81
Veterinary Informatics and Epidemiology   82
Diagnostics   83
Point of care analysers   83
Acute phase proteins   83
Ultrasound and endoscopy   84
Collaboration with the Moredun   85
Research Institute
Veterinary Diagnostic Services   86
Commercialism and technology transfer   86
Conclusions   87

Chapter 5:
Bricks and Mortar

The Veterinary Hospital at Garscube   90
Garscube House   91
Clinical, pre and para - clinical facilities   93
The Byres   93
Cochno Estate   94
Netherton Farm   94
The Small Animal Hospital   95
Planning for further major developments   96
The Weipers Centre for Equine Welfare   97
New Small Animal Hospital   98
Scottish Centre for Production Animal   100
Health and Food Safety
The Research Environment   101
Wellcome/MRC Laboratories for   101
Experimental Parasitology
The Wellcome Surgical Institute   101
The pre- and para- clinical building   102
(Phase I) at Garscube
Research in the Phase I building   103
The Leukaemia Research Fund Virus   103
Centre
The Henry Wellcome Building for   104
Comparative Medical Sciences
Looking to the future   104
The Centre for Virus Research   104
Teaching and student areas   105
Lecture facilities and practical classes   105
The James Herriot Library   105
The GUVMA hut   106
The GLASS project   106
Conclusions   107

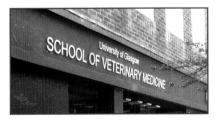

Glasgow Vet School

Chapter 6:
Glasgow Vets Overseas

Early Days   111
Veterinary services and research in   111
West Africa
Veterinary Schools in East Africa: 112
1963 and onwards
New international research laboratories   114
1970- 1980s
International Laboratory for Research on   114
Animal Diseases, Nairobi Kenya
The International Trypanotolerance   116
Centre in the Gambia
Trypanosomiasis   117
Trypanosomiasis control strategies   118
The use of trypanocidal drugs   118
The use of genetic resistance   120
Human African trypanosomiasis   121
Return to The Gambia   122
Calum's Road   122
Donkey football   122
Control of other enzootic, epizootic   123
and zoonotic diseases
Primary health care technology transfer: 124
bovine mastitis
Reflections on the African diaspora: 124
an everlasting bond

Afterword   127
Appendices   129
Heads of Glasgow Veterinary School   129
Honorary Degrees and Fellowships   130
Staff list   131
Emeritus, Honorary and Visiting   134
Appointees
Memorial lectures   135
Photograph legends   137
Abbreviations   138
References   139

Chapter One

The McCall Years 1862 -1915

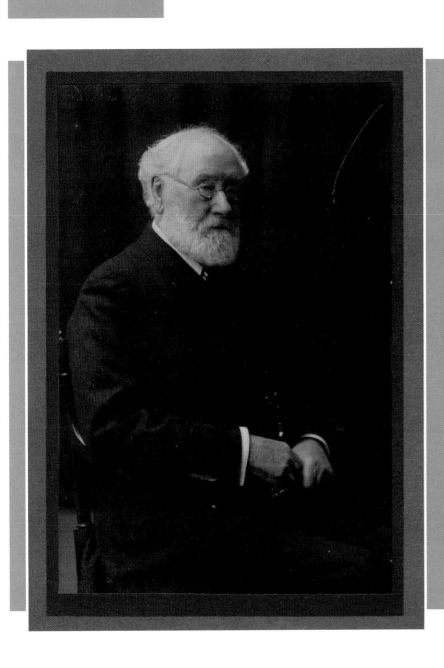

The Beginning

The Glasgow Veterinary College was founded in 1862 by James McCall, Fellow of the Royal College of Veterinary Surgeons, one hundred years after the establishment of the first Veterinary School in Europe by Claude Bourgelat in Lyons.[1] With a career spanning over fifty years as Principal, the early history of the College is closely interwoven with James McCall: the welfare and development of the College was very much a private and personal venture and a lifetime achievement.

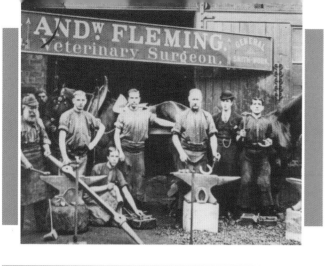

Andrew Fleming Veterinary Premises, Rutherglen 1890s

James McCall, founder and first Principal

James McCall was born in Ayrshire in 1834 at Newton-on-Ayr. His father ran a transport business as a carrier between Glasgow and Ayr where McCall gained his early experience in working with horses. He was educated at Wallacetown and Ayr Academies and later apprenticed to a lawyer's office in Ayr on his father's wishes. However his legal career did not last very long and he became superintendent of the horse department with Messrs Pickford & Co, the railway contractors in London, caring for as many as a thousand horses. While in London he became interested in the study of the medical treatment of the horse and decided that he wanted to become a veterinarian.[4] He had by this time introduced the use of the nosebag for long journeys thus alleviating cases of colic by allowing the horse to feed intermittently through the day rather than gorging at night.[5]

At that time, the only formal training available in Scotland was through the Edinburgh Veterinary College, now known as the Royal (Dick) School of Veterinary Studies, which was established in 1823 by William Dick, the pioneer of veterinary education in Scotland.

In Glasgow, the first move to provide veterinary education had been made when Josiah Cheetham, who had also qualified from the Edinburgh Veterinary College, was appointed to the chair in Veterinary Surgery in 1832 in the Medical School of the Andersonian Institution.

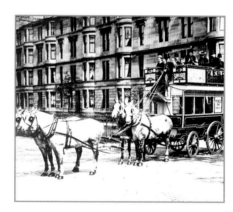

Horse drawn bus 1890s

He remained for six months. He was succeeded by John Stewart in 1834 who had studied in Edinburgh and London. He remained until 1840 then left Glasgow for Sydney, Australia where he contributed much to the development of veterinary and agricultural science, and advised the Government of New South Wales on agricultural policy.[6]

McCall studied for two years in Edinburgh, qualifying in 1857 with the diploma of the Highland and Agricultural Society of Scotland. The Edinburgh Veterinary College was situated on Clyde Street where the Saint Andrew's Square bus station now stands. The curriculum at this time consisted of two sessions or academic years from October/November followed by a single oral examination in April.[7] The fee was 16 guineas (plus one guinea for the library) for which the 'pupil has the privilege of attending the lectures as long as he pleases; of witnessing Mr Dick's practice which is pretty extensive; of attending the lectures of several eminent medical men; and there is no additional expense incurred for the diploma'.

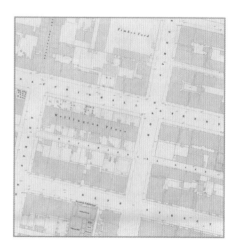

Sauchiehall Lane

1862

Glasgow Veterinary College founded by James McCall.

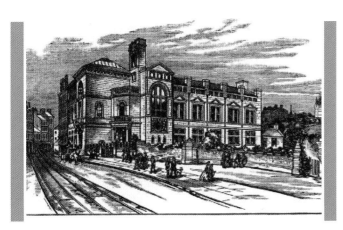

Founded by the will of John Anderson, Professor of Natural Philosophy at the University of Glasgow, Anderson's Institution was established in 1796.[8] It became known as Anderson's University in 1828 and Anderson's College in 1877. In 1887, its medical school, from which David Livingstone had graduated, became independent and was incorporated as Anderson's College Medical School. It finally was amalgamated with the Faculty of Medicine of the University of Glasgow in 1947.

The rest of the College merged with other institutions to become the main component of the Glasgow and West of Scotland Technical College which later became the University of Strathclyde in 1964. Anderson's Institution was originally located in John Street but moved to George Street. In 1889 the Medical School buildings relocated to Dumbarton Road close to the Western Infirmary[9] and they now house the University of Glasgow International College.[10]

Anderson's College

Early Days

After six months in a country practice at Symington in Ayrshire, McCall was offered the Chair of Anatomy by William Dick and returned to Edinburgh to teach anatomy and physiology for two sessions.[11] His predecessor John Gamgee had left to start a new veterinary school in Edinburgh.[12] Gamgee had been particularly interested in the control of infectious diseases in animals and had views which were incompatible with Dick's.[13] Gamgee's opinions were spectacularly vindicated when a devastating outbreak of cattle plague (rinderpest) occurred in Britain in 1865, introduced by cattle imported from Latvia. Dick believed that the disease could be treated, which proved completely unsuccessful. By contrast, Gamgee and McCall advocated accurate diagnosis, with quarantine and slaughter of affected animals, a policy that was ultimately successful in eradicating the disease and which in due course set a pattern for the control of other serious infectious diseases of animals.

In 1859, when only twenyfive years old, McCall returned to Glasgow and opened a practice in Hope Street, near which in 56 Sauchiehall Lane in a small shoeing forge, he gave a course of lectures to a number of Edinburgh students living in Glasgow.

Three students came for an hour in the evening to hear McCall lecture to increase their zoological knowledge.[14] Formal classes began in 1862 and ten students enrolled; five were intending professionals and five were not. McCall lectured for three hours each day on anatomy, physiology and surgery, and the students attended the materia medica and chemistry classes of Dr Martin and Dr Penny in Anderson's University.[15]

In 1863, McCall moved his practice to larger premises at 397 Parliamentary Road near the Caledonian Railway Company's stables. Lectures and demonstrations continued in the new premises which had been fitted with stables, a shoeing forge, a hospital and a loose box. McCall had a room on the ground floor as a surgery. In 1862, he had applied to the RCVS for a Charter for the establishment of the College as a centre for training for the examinations, at that time conducted by the Royal College. Both the London Veterinary College and the Dick Vet in Edinburgh vigorously opposed the application. However, the School had its supporters, including Lord Lister – who had carried out some of his early experiments with antiseptics in the original College premises in Parliamentary Road.[16] (It is the 100th anniversary of the death of Lister in 2012).

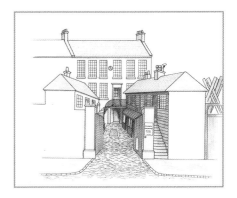

Premises at Parliamentary Road

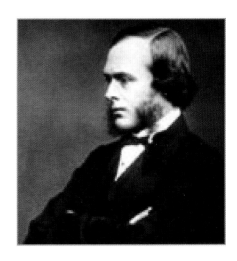

Lord Lister

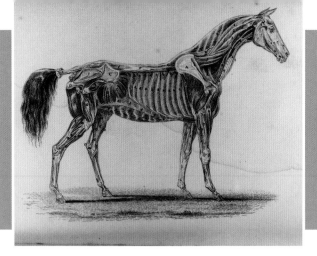

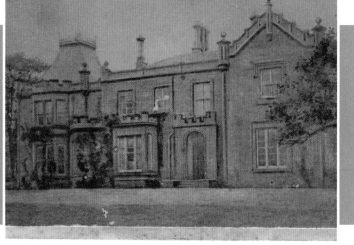

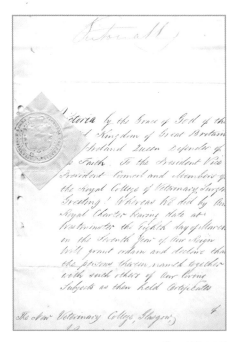

Royal Warrant

Professor George Armatage was among the College's distinguished staff at this time. He maintained the need for longer training of veterinary students, a thorough set of examinations and the maintenance of proper selection procedures (all of which continue to be under constant scrutiny even today!).

Armatage also was the author of 'The Thermometer as an Aid to Diagnosis in Veterinary Medicine'.

He claimed that the clinical thermometer was a more 'infallible test of approaching contagious disease, its gradual progress in intensity, or the more welcome approach of convalescence'.[17]

Following the application by McCall, a Royal Warrant was granted by Queen Victoria on 2nd June 1863 for 'the new Veterinary College, Glasgow' recognising its teaching for the examinations of the RCVS and admitting its students who passed that examination to all the privileges granted to the members of the RCVS. The first graduates, Messrs A Anderson, T Campbell and P Findlay, qualified in April 1865.

From these modest beginnings, the College steadily progressed and the number of students attending had increased from ten to fiftytwo students by 1874 with the exception of a small dip in admissions in the 1865-1866 sessions when an entrance exam for students was introduced. The majority of the students were attracted from the West of Scotland and Ireland who chose the nearer destination of Glasgow rather than that of Edinburgh.

Over the years the veterinary course changed in both content and duration. Up until 1876 the course occupied only two years. However, in 1876 this was lengthened to three years with an examination at the end of each year.

In 1895 the course was extended to four years and it was not until thirtyseven years later in 1932 when it finally became a five year course which it has remained.'[18,19]

In addition to his teaching duties, Principal McCall undertook many other activities. He was interested in the promotion of public health measures and held a number of public appointments including 'Inspector to the Glasgow Corporation' under the Diseases of Animals Act which stated that veterinary surgeons, in addition to medical officers or sanitary inspectors, could act as meat inspectors.[20,21] Through his influence, Glasgow had the distinction of being the first city in the UK to introduce meat market inspection and the licensing of city dairies. He was consulted by the Veterinary Department of the Ministry of Agriculture under the Diseases of Animals Acts, and the Tuberculosis Order.

He acted as veterinary surgeon to a number of railway contractors whose large numbers of horses supplied clinical teaching material for his students.[22] McCall was also a farmer and had properties in Garrowhill, Carmunnock; Flemington, Cambuslang; Blairtummock Easterhouse (Blairtummock House is now restored and a business and conference centre[23]); and latterly at Burnhead and Woodend, Kilsyth. He achieved distinction as a breeder of Ayrshire cattle and Clydesdale horses.[24] His grandson Stewart Johnson McCall later introduced Clydesdales to Australia in 1920.[25]

Principal McCall realised the importance of the RCVS in maintaining standards in veterinary education and played an active role in the College, becoming President in 1890-1891. He was awarded the John Henry Steel medal by the College in 1899.[26]

1863

Royal Charter granted to James McCall establishing Glasgow Veterinary College.

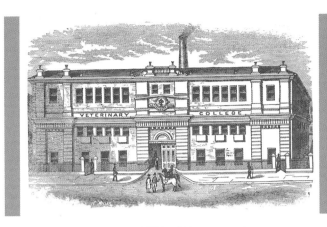

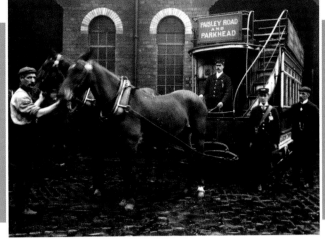

Move to Buccleuch Street

By 1873, Principal McCall learned that a water pumping station, originally built for the new Glasgow water supply from Loch Katrine and later converted to stables for the Glasgow Corporation tramway system, was available at 82 - 83 Buccleuch Street in Garnethill.[27] The premises could provide the accommodation required for the development of the College.

The quadrangular three-storey building with a central yard covered by a glass roof was reconstructed into laboratories and classrooms and equipped with a shoeing forge and stables. There was also surplus space which was let as a stable and dairy. The space was formally opened by Professor Knox on the 28th October 1874, who claimed that the premises 'when finished will be the most complete for the training of veterinary surgeons in Scotland if not Great Britain'[28].

The course at this time consisted of only two years with no formal entry requirements, though Professor James Weir, FRCVS who taught physiology at Parliamentary Road related that intending students were submitted to a general intelligence interview which included a test in reading passages from the 'Glasgow Herald' and commenting on the subject matter.[29]

Histology and botany were added to the curriculum and a summer session of two months was introduced.

The early members of the Glasgow College staff included Professor Fordie in medicine and Professor James Macqueen in surgery who was succeeded by his brother, Professor AS Macqueen. Professor James Macqueen studied in Glasgow in 1877 and stayed on with Principal McCall as house surgeon and later as Lecturer in Anatomy, Materia Medica and Surgery. In 1888 he was invited to teach at the Royal Veterinary College in London and lectured there on many subjects. He was appointed to its chair in surgery in 1895 and was a pioneer of equine abdominal surgery. He was an examiner for many years and held positions including president within the National Medical Veterinary Association, forerunner of the British Veterinary Association.[30,31]

Student numbers continued to increase and one hundred and fortythree students had enrolled at the Glasgow College by 1894. Towards the end of the 19th Century and beginning of the 20th Century, staff included Professor Stephen Cook in chemistry and Professor King in botany. They were succeeded by Professor Scott Elliot and Professor AN McAlpine and two of Professor McCall's sons, Dr James McCall and Professor John R McCall. The latter returned from the First World War in 1918 to the Chair of Materia Medica and Pharmacy.

Professor James F Murphy, a versatile Irishman, taught anatomy from 1897 up to his death at the end of the war. Professor David Imrie from Bishopbriggs taught medicine and surgery for a number of years after 1918.[32]

Lecture notes 1886

The fees at that time for the three year veterinary course were £16 for the first year, £18 for the second and £20 for the third.[33]

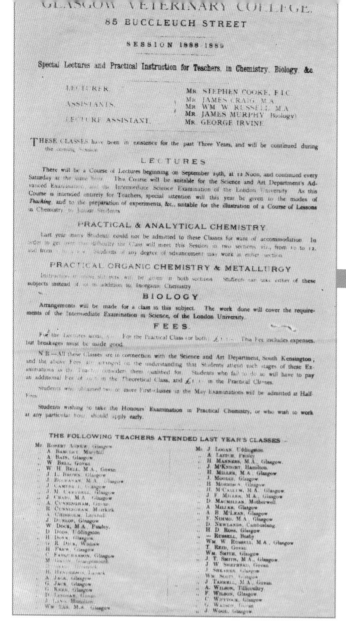

Poster for session 1888-1889 Special Lectures and Practical Instruction for teachers

A Glasgow student who formed a long and close association with the College was Hugh Begg, FRCVS from Hamilton who graduated in 1887. He was the first holder of a post as a County Veterinary Inspector in Scotland, in Lanark.

Another notable student was John Gilruth, 1893 graduate, who earned worldwide recognition for his work in New Zealand where he was the first Government Veterinary Surgeon and then in Australia where he was Administrator of the Northern Territory and went on to become first chief of the New Division of Animal Health within the Council for Scientific and Industrial Research.[34]

A student who qualified from the Glasgow Vet College in 1886 recalled (in 1945) that 'Practice was hard in those days – driving all day and half the night in all weathers in gigs and dogcarts. The present day graduate does not know what hard work and exposure is.' Many cruel operations were performed as chloroform and anaesthetics were unknown in veterinary practice when he began.

He also describes his final year examiners in horse and cattle pathology as 'great toffs appearing in toppers with morning coats or frock coats and shaped trousers'.[35]

After 1894, student numbers decreased. This was thought to be related to the establishment of the higher entrance qualifications and the longer four year course which also added to the teaching responsibilities of the College. In addition, the opening of the Dublin school in 1895 deprived Glasgow of one-third of its intake.[36]

The day to day work of the practising veterinarian was largely concerned with 'keeping the wheels of the transport industry turning' in the care of the horse. In Glasgow, as in any large city, horses supplied power for public transport, deliveries for docks and railways, vessels on canals, the funeral cortege and farm work. Additionally, the army relied on horse drawn transport.[37]

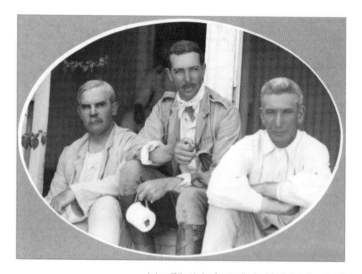

John Gilruth in Australia in 1912 (on the right) with Josiah Thomas and Sir Walter Barttelot

1949
Amalgamation of the Vet College with the University with William Weipers as Director.

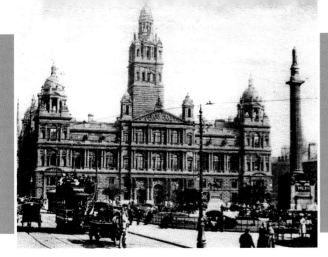

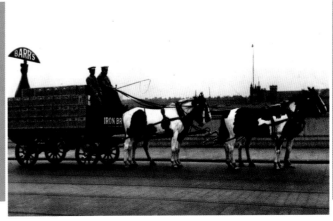

'What are we about in Glasgow for the cure of diseases among horses'

An article about the College in the Southern Press in 1900 asked 'What are we about in Glasgow for the cure of diseases among horses'. The journalist was given a tour of the College by Professor Murphy and found evidence of 'work of a busy lifetime' in Principal McCall's museum. For example, he saw dried dissections and wax facsimiles of abnormal subjects in glass cases showing muscles, blood vessels and nerves; illustrations peculiar to the lower animals such as foot and mouth disease, glanders, pleuropneumonia, anthrax..; parts of animals preserved in jars of alcohol showing diseased conditions of specific internal organs; a horse's skull showing a cleft palate; specimens of the teeth illustrating the age of the horse and other domestic animals. He also noted that the College dealt with all sorts of animals. 'There you have a cyclopean lamb, there you have a sheltie in situ with the heart, principal blood vessels and many of the chief muscles displayed'. A Shetland pony had been treated by McCall for a broken leg. The pony had to have an amputation below the hock. McCall had then made a wooden leg and leather stocking with the hoof attached to the shoe so that the pony could move freely. The journalist was impressed with his findings, 'A horse with a wooden leg is as rare as a dog with false teeth'.

The journalist was also impressed with Professor Murphy's collections. 'He had specimens illustrating the animal kingdom from the protozoa to man; many singular anomalies preserved in alcohol and skeletons of various animals; a lemur as an example of the art of taxidermy and most uniquely, a large collection of parasites of the lower animals.'[38]

Professor Murphy wrote to the 'Evening Times' in 1909 regarding the closure of Glasgow Zoo. Principal McCall and Professor Murphy had treated some of the animals, including a baby elephant with a broken leg, a lion with a mangled tail and a small monkey whose finger had been chewed by a chimpanzee.[39] Professor Murphy thought the zoo should be saved as it was beneficial to the veterinary and agricultural students for education in zoology, comparative anatomy, pathology and medicine. He also thought it could be useful for the Army veterinarian if he needed to treat a camel or an elephant. However, the zoo was closed in 1909 and the animal collection was dispersed.[40]

Glasgow Veterinary College Incorporated as a Public Institution

Principal McCall realised that survival of his College lay with its incorporation as a public body and its recognition as a Central Institution with a board of governors.

This was achieved in 1909, when it was recognised as a Central Institution by the Scottish Education Department and a government grant was made available to help with the purchase and maintenance of the College. Members of the board included representatives from the University of Glasgow, the Faculty of Physicians and Surgeons Glasgow (now the Royal College of Physicians and Surgeons of Glasgow), the Corporation of Glasgow, the Education Authority of Glasgow and various County Councils in the area of the College at that time.[41] With the £5083 raised by the Governors and a Government grant of £5000, the College buildings were purchased from McCall who continued to hold his post as Principal.[42] During Principal McCall's long leadership of the College, nearly five hundred students graduated many making important contributions to veterinary science, colonial administration, research and scientific work and in teaching. Five of McCall's sons followed him into his profession.

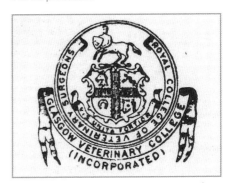

Crest

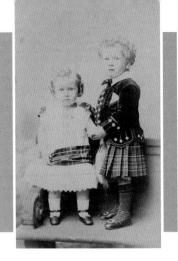
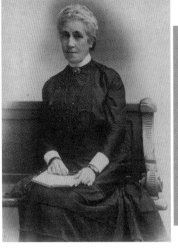
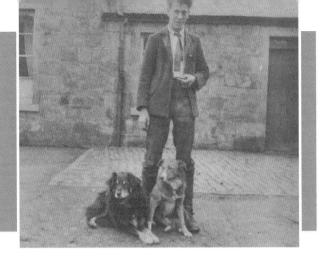

McCall's sons - Stewart and George

McCall's wife - Clementina

McCall's son - Stewart

McCall family history

Principal McCall combined a busy professional life with a full domestic one. He was married twice and brought up seven daughters and nine sons. His first wife Williamina Aitken Walker was from a well-known Glasgow family of that time, the Walkers of Lethamhill.

McCall's second wife, Clementina Stuart Johnston, was the daughter of Reverend Dr Johnston, Minister of Cambuslang. McCall's sons who followed him into the veterinary profession held various positions at home and abroad; his eldest son Dr James McIntosh McCall, FRCVS of the Board of Agriculture and Fisheries was also a Doctor of Medicine; Professor John R McCall of the Glasgow College and head of Veterinary Sciences at the Scottish Agricultural College 'his deputy in many aspects'[43]; George, Frederick and David McCall, Members of the RCVS who held important positions in South Africa; Mr Stewart McCall, eldest son of his second family was a Director of Agriculture in Nyasaland.[44]

If any of his seven daughters had wanted to become vets, they would have had to wait until 1919 for the passing of the Sex Disqualification (Removal) Act when all of the veterinary colleges began to accept female students, with the exception of the Royal (Dick) Veterinary College, which gave its excuse as the lack of a suitable lavatory.[45]

Principal McCall continued to direct the affairs of the College and worked up to five weeks before his death at the age of 81. His funeral took place on 4 November 1915, attended by many mourners, including staff from the Veterinary College and Glasgow Corporation officials. Five of his sons were unable to attend as they were on active service. He was buried in the Glasgow Necropolis.[46] His brother Andrew McCall was also buried there. His memorial, a Celtic cross was the first commission of a young architect, Charles Rennie McIntosh.[47]

Who would have thought that one man could have had such vision and foresight? James McCall over the course of approximately fiftyfive years developed the course and fabric of what was to become the Glasgow Veterinary College. From its humble beginnings in a small shoeing forge in Sauchiehall Lane, where he lectured to three students, to its premises in Buccleuch Street, McCall was integral to the foundation of the Veterinary School in Glasgow with hundreds of students graduating and shaping the future of the profession.

Without a man like McCall, with such a vision for the future, dedication to veterinary science and insight one can only wonder whether we would ever have had the good fortune to celebrate the existence of 150 years of the Glasgow Veterinary School.

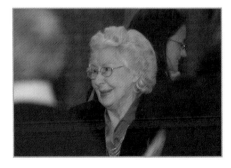

Theresa Anderson at inaugural memorial lecture for her grandfather James McCall 2008

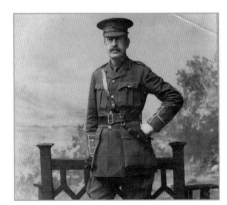

McCall's son - John

1950

The bovine lungworm vaccine produced.

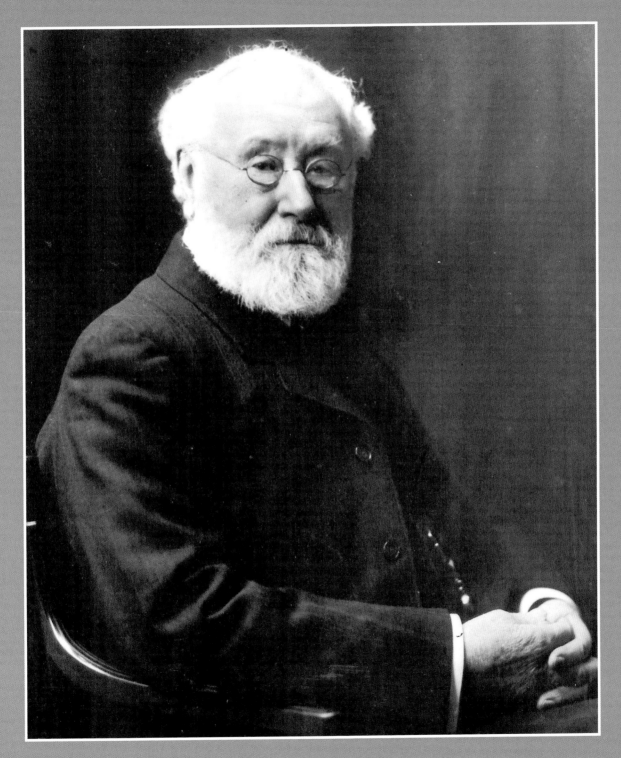

James McCall

Chapter Two

The Pre-University College
1915-1949

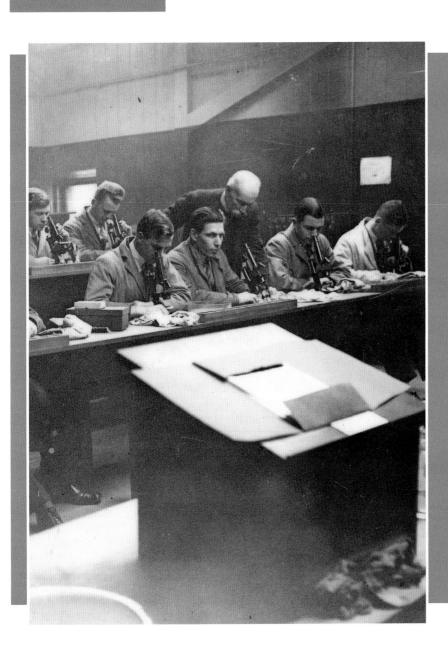

New Era, New Principals

Between 1909 and 1920, enrolments increased from fortytwo to seventythree students, although the numbers had decreased between 1914 and 1918, reflecting the effects of war.[48] Post-war, many students were ex-army, supported by grants and seemed more mature and sophisticated.[49]

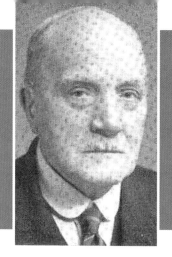
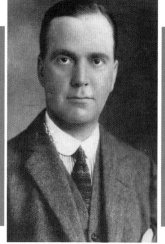
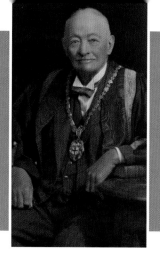
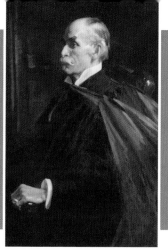

Principal Hugh Begg (1915-1917)

Following Principal McCall's death in 1915, Hugh Begg, former student, house surgeon and Board member was asked to serve as interim Principal. Begg acted in this capacity until 1917 when Sidney Gaiger, who was also Professor of Pathology, was appointed Principal by the Board.[50]

Principal Sidney Gaiger (1917-1922)

Professor Gaiger had spent time abroad in Chile and in India at the Mucktesar research station. While abroad he developed glanders, (an infectious disease of equines which can also infect humans)[51], and had his left arm amputated as a result.

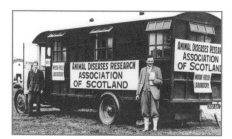

1928 Animal Diseases Research Association (now Moredun Foundation) mobile laboratory

Early Research in Buccleuch Street

Professor Gaiger was encouraged by the Governors to embark on an ambitious programme of research, mainly into the diseases of sheep. This was the main veterinary research work carried out in Scotland at that time. A bacteriology laboratory at the College was created consisting of a research lab, histology room, house for small experimental animals and accommodation for sheep. Much of the grant came from the Board of Agriculture of Scotland.[52]

From his research, Principal Gaiger developed a vaccine to prevent braxy in sheep, a disease caused by *Clostridium septicum*. He was also interested in other diseases such as 'trembling' and liver fluke. He held the post as Principal until 1922 when he was appointed joint director along with his assistant Mr Thomas Dalling of the newly formed Animal Diseases Research Association which established the Moredun Institute in Edinburgh. This marked the beginning of a long association of Glasgow staff with the Institute.[53]

Principal Arthur Whitehouse (1922-1944)

Later in 1922 Dr Arthur Wildman Whitehouse was appointed Principal and Professor of Anatomy. A popular choice, he was born in Brighton and studied the classics before heading to the American West to run a large ranch where he bred and reared cattle extensively. However, when the enterprise met with hard times, he studied for a veterinary degree in Toronto. He had taught anatomy in Fort Collins Veterinary College, Colorado but went to France as a Veterinary Officer when war broke out in 1914 returning to teaching in 1918 after the armistice. He came to the Glasgow College in 1922 as a Director of Studies. As his qualification was not recognised by the RCVS, he spent a year in Liverpool qualifying as MRCVS.[54] He then had to sit his second professional examination alongside his Glasgow students having spent the year teaching them anatomy.[55]

1951

Chairs of Veterinary Surgery and Veterinary Pathology established.

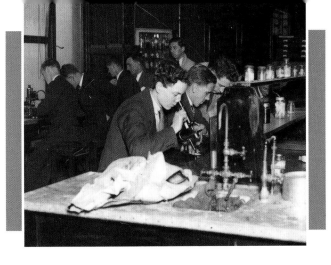

Buccleuch Street Lab

Uncertain times – the Constable Report

This was an uncertain time for Whitehouse and the College; although enrolments were increasing, student fees had not been collected during 1914-1918. In 1920, the Governors planned a public appeal for new buildings which would cost around £30,000. It was not launched as there were indications that official government policy was that only one veterinary college was necessary in Scotland and that resources should be concentrated on the one centred in Edinburgh.

A Departmental Committee was appointed in 1924 under Lord Constable 'To consider and advise regarding the general organisation and finance of agricultural research in Scotland'. The Constable Report formally recommended that two veterinary colleges were unnecessary and that the grant of state assistance to Glasgow should be discontinued. Not all on the committee agreed and Mr Walter Elliot, MP submitted a minority report. Indeed, Sir Robert Greig of the Board of Agriculture suggested the number of schools should be increased to three, with a college situated in Aberdeen.

The state grant to Glasgow was withdrawn in 1925 and not re-established for another twenty years. A public meeting was held in Glasgow to protest against the withdrawal but to no avail. An article in the 'Glasgow Herald' stated that 'the city's Parliamentary representatives on both sides of the House have shown themselves united in defence of the Veterinary College in a degree which has not manifested itself on almost any other public question… To ask the Glasgow College to close down and to cause its students to travel to Edinburgh for tuition that is already provided in a manner that is to the credit of the Glasgow College is surely a strange step to take in the name of either national economy or educational efficiency.'

The Glasgow College survived these very difficult circumstances due to the efforts of Professor John Glaister of the University of Glasgow, Chairman of the Board of Governors, Principal Whitehouse, James Austin, the Secretary of the College and the small group of enthusiastic part time and full time teachers.

Student fees accounted for 80 percent of the total income of the College. The remainder was derived from local authorities. Economies were made with, at times, Principal Whitehouse as the only full time staff member, while free tuition in clinical subjects to final year students was given by veterinary surgeons in the West of Scotland. Students showed their loyalty and support by organising collections on behalf of the College funds.

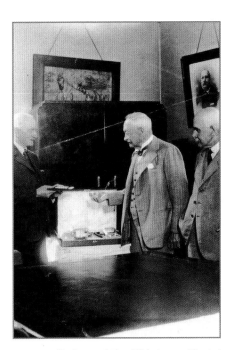

Professor Arthur Whitehouse (Centre)

Whitehouse was involved in the framing of the extended five year course and the standardising of examinations with the RCVS. The Glasgow students attained high passes comparable to other Colleges, which was testimony to the efficient training at the College despite the testing times. Principal Whitehouse was justly proud of the College's achievements.[57,58]

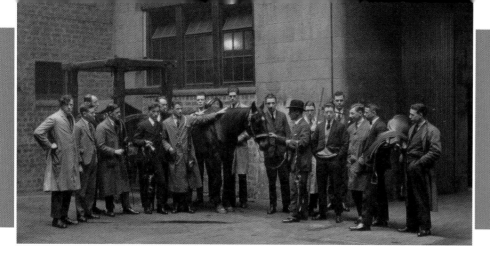

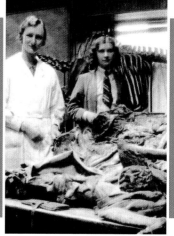

The Loveday Committee

In 1937, the Loveday Committee was appointed by the Government to report on the essential needs of the facilities for training veterinarians in the UK. The first report set out the views of the Committee: 'The system of education and conditions in the Schools are unsatisfactory. The basic sciences are in general not adequately taught. The prescribed courses of study concentrate on animal sickness and treat the maintenance of health altogether too lightly. Attention is focussed too completely on the curative aspect to the neglect of the preventive: animal husbandry in its wider sense – that vital section of veterinary education – is not stressed. The farm animal receives too little consideration relatively to that given to the horse, dog and cat. The particular system of external examination in force must tend to deflect teaching into channels prejudicial to sound education. At the Schools, the teaching staff are inadequate and in many instances stipends are low and out of all proportion to the responsibilities which the posts carry; proper facilities for clinical training and for the practical side of animal husbandry are everywhere lacking; under the pressure of financial stringency students have been admitted in excessive numbers, with the result that the classrooms and laboratories are overcrowded; and the teachers have neither time nor facilities for research'.

They considered that the 'one portal system' of entry to the profession, registration by the RCVS should be maintained. Other recommendations included farm pupillage, the provision of field stations and large animal hospitals and a period of 'seeing practice'. They put forward a revised curriculum for the five year course of study: a three year veterinary science degree course within a university and two years of clinical training at an existing veterinary school.

They also referred to the problem of training 'town boys' or 'suburbanites' as compared with the sons of farmers and did not see a great role for women practitioners, training them only for 'work among dogs and cats'.

With the outbreak of war in 1939, the Loveday Committee's recommended actions were put on hold until peace was restored.[59]

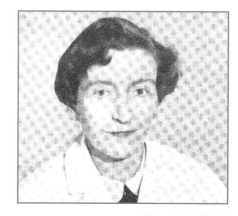

Helen 'Nellie' Smith

First Scottish women veterinary students

During Dr Whitehouse's nineteen years as Principal, he oversaw many changes. The Glasgow College was first of the two Scottish veterinary schools to accept women students. The first female students Marion Stewart and Gerda Gillies enrolled in 1925, followed in 1926 by (Agnes) Maud Catchpole and Phyllis Wilson.

By 1940, eighteen women students had been admitted. Conditions were primitive. The women entered through a door next to the office of Dr Whitehouse. There was no place to study though they had use of the common room on the second floor where the janitor Mr Stoker and his wife and daughter sold rolls, sandwiches and teas. Mary Duff, who enrolled in 1931, recalled that 'tuition was scrappy and it amazed us all that anyone got through'. However the first women graduates remembered their time with affection and not as a time of discrimination. They were sometimes excluded from male social events but not from pranks such as 'meat fights' in the anatomy laboratories.

During the inter-war years, 1918-1938, jobs were hard to come by particularly for women. Most women went into small animal practice. Marion Stewart who graduated in 1930 and was the first women to be registered MRCVS in Scotland,[60] worked in London and published details of her cases in the Veterinary Record.

1954

The new veterinary school, the building of which began in 1950, opens at Garscube.

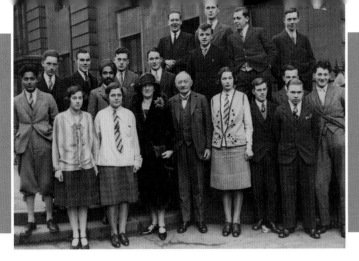

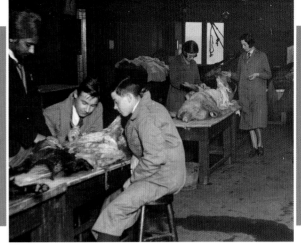

She went into practice with another Glasgow vet, Muriel Shinnie. She continued her work with small animals when she went to Rhodesia in 1945.

Going abroad to find work was a well-worn path by many female Scottish graduates who found it difficult to break into a male dominated profession.

Maud Catchpole also ran a small animal practice in London before returning home to help her father manage a silver fox farm. She received support from Burroughs Wellcome to study the treatment of leptospirosis in silver fox cubs.

Two of these early female graduates achieved distinction. Helen Mitchell (married name Helen Smith), worked as an assistant to Dr Whitehouse in anatomy after her graduation in 1933 and succeeded him on his retirement. Affectionately known as Nellie Smith, she was later promoted to senior lecturership in 1955 and in 1958 was the first woman to join the University Senate. She also played a large part in designing the new anatomy department at Garscube. She is remembered as a 'superb gross anatomist who could balance her cigarette neatly on its end when she needed both hands to make a point'. The cigarette smoke could also disguise the smell of the formalin and other smells in the anatomy laboratory which could be a shock to the young veterinary students.

THE GLASGOW VETERINARY COLLEGE
Incorporated

PROFESSIONAL STAFF

SALARY SCALES

JUNIOR LECTURERS	-	£485 x £25 - £825.
SENIOR LECTURERS	-	£680 x £30 - £1,100.
PROFESSORS	-	£1,350.

Scales for Women - 80% of above.

Salary scales 1949

Eudo Sime (married name Cockrill) graduated in 1937. In 1943 she became the first female vet to be appointed to the Field Service in the Ministry of Agriculture and Fisheries.

After the war, she and her husband, also a vet, worked overseas with the Food and Agriculture Association (FAO). While in Rome, she taught in the American Overseas School and studied for her DVM at Pisa.[61]

In the 1940s, after the end of the Second World War, women again faced difficulties in gaining entry to the College as many places were taken by young men returning from the armed forces. Margaret Cameron, a farmer's daughter, succeeded in her second attempt in 1947. Six girls were in her first year, the most that had ever been in Glasgow. She went on to devote her life to small animal practice, spending much of her career as a principal in a veterinary practice in Dundee. Her experience gained at the free clinic run by the junior staff of Buccleuch Street was invaluable and in all her years of practice 'very rarely did she meet a client who specifically requested to see a male veterinary surgeon'.[62]

By 1937, the total of number of both male and female enrolments had increased to 282 students. Most of these students (223) came from the areas within close proximity to the College. The others came from areas further away in the UK and overseas such as South Africa, India, Israel, West Indies and Burma.

The Governors considered that the location of the College in Glasgow contributed to national interests due to the livestock industry within the area served and that all students who qualified could be placed within the profession.[63,64]

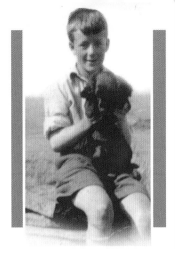

From Jim Wight's biography of his father Alf Wight… A red setter named Don, an article in 'Meccano Magazine' about being a vet, and a talk by the Principal of the Veterinary College, Dr Whitehouse, at his school, Hillhead High School when Alf Wight was thirteen, all influenced his desire to become a veterinary surgeon. Alf Wight was educated at the Glasgow Veterinary College and qualified MRCVS in 1939 (after six and a half years which was regarded then as relatively quick compared to the time taken by some semi-permanent students). He regarded his time spent at the College in that 'seedy old building' as some of the happiest years of his life. In his biography of his father, Jim Wight describes a session at one of the infamous Vet School dances which took place on most Friday nights. Alf regularly attended these throbbing sessions.

His friend Alex Taylor had asked if he could come along although his mother had heard that it could be a bit rough. However as it was Fresher's Night, extra spice was added. The night started out in a Glasgow public house. Following the consumption of much beer and whisky, the students tried to gatecrash the dance and in the melee Alex was punched on the chin and knocked out. In a burst of inspiration, as the dance was held on the upper floor of the College and several long boxes from an earlier delivery of microscopes and new lab equipment filled with wood shavings were sitting in the yard below, he and his friends dragged Alex downstairs. However there was a snag, a number of the boxes were already comfortably occupied by inebriated students sleeping peacefully. However, an empty one was found for Alex and the friends returned to the dance floor.[65]

Young Alf

Alf Wight 1939 graduate, 'Glasgow's most famous vet'

The James Herriot Library at Glasgow Veterinary School is named in honour of James Alfred Wight (1916-1995), a Glasgow Veterinary College graduate of 1939 who became famous under the pseudonym James Herriot for his books of stories about the life of a country vet.[66]

After a short spell working in Sunderland, Alf Wight joined a practice in Thirsk in rural North Yorkshire, and began to write about his experiences in later life. 'If Only They Could Talk' was published thirty years after his graduation in 1969. Although initially it was a struggle to find a publisher, his first book was a great success and was followed by six more books, two films and a popular television series, 'All Creatures Great and Small'. The author was appointed OBE in 1979. A biography of Alf Wight was published by his son Jim Wight, who is a 1966 Glasgow veterinary graduate. Alf Wight took the pseudonym 'James Herriot' to avoid breaking RCVS regulations at the time regarding advertising. He chose the name after attending a football match in which the Scotland international player Jim Herriot played in goal for Birmingham City;[67] there were no vets in the RCVS Register with this surname.

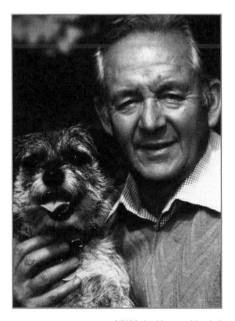

Alf Wight (James Herriot)

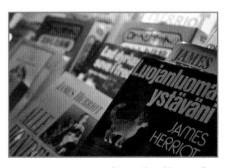

International best sellers

Eddie Straiton 1940 graduate, larger than life TV vet

Eddie Straiton (1917 – 2004), from Clydebank and a 1940 graduate was a contemporary of Alf Wight and lifelong friend. A flamboyant character, he was regarded as a great all - rounder of the veterinary profession and the original 'TV Vet'. He started a regular television feature in 1957 giving advice to farmers on animal health and welfare on 'Farming Today'. He went on to broadcast widely and to write a series of popular veterinary text books while slotting all of his activities into his busy practice life in Staffordshire. He was awarded an OBE at the age of eighty for his lifetime crusades on behalf of animal welfare.[68,69]

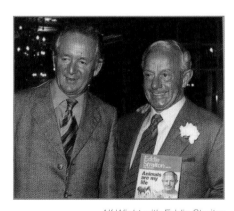

Alf Wight with Eddie Straiton

1954
Cochno Estate purchased.

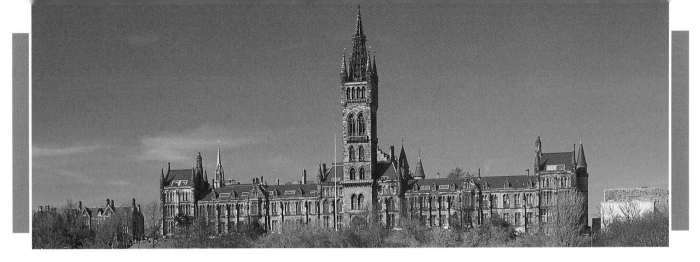

The Loveday Report revisited 1944

The second Loveday Report was published in 1944. The Loveday Committee was asked to review its recommendations of its first report in 1937 in light of Government plans to maintain a healthy and well balanced agriculture after the war. The second report recognised the need for considerable expansion and improvement in veterinary schools and recommended that training should be carried out in universities.[70] Conditions were set by the report: financial assistance would be provided by the state; the degree in veterinary science or medicine awarded by the University would be a registrable qualification for membership of the RCVS; and the University would have control over the courses and the examinations.[71]

When the University of Glasgow showed willingness to undertake responsibility for veterinary education, the Department of Agriculture re-established its grant in 1945. The Board of Governors formally handed over the College to the University Court in October 1945 although the need for further negotiations meant that unity was not established until 1949.[72] The Veterinary Surgeons Act in 1948 set up the current system under which veterinary degrees awarded by the Universities of Bristol, Cambridge, Edinburgh, Glasgow, Liverpool and London were recognised by the RCVS.[73]

The last Principals of the Old College; Donald Campbell (1945 -1946) and Albert Forsyth (1946 - 1949)

Dr Whitehouse was Principal until 1944. He was succeeded by Donald Campbell as Principal and Professor of Medicine. When he died suddenly in 1946, Albert Forsyth, who had been a practitioner in Staffordshire until he was injured, was then engaged as Principal on a three year contract. He later moved on to a senior position in the United Nations Food and Agriculture Organisation.

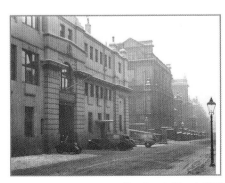

Buccleuch Street 1953

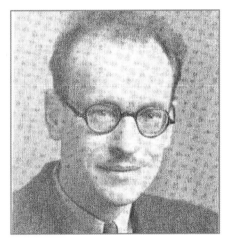

Donald Campbell

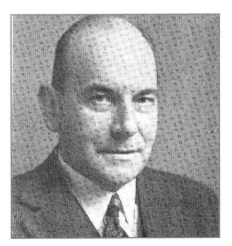

Albert Forsyth

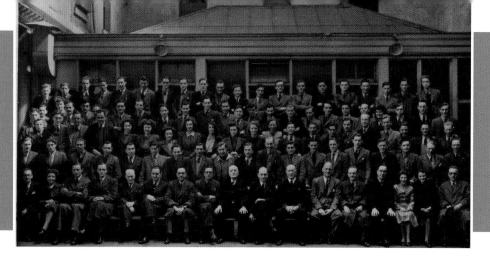

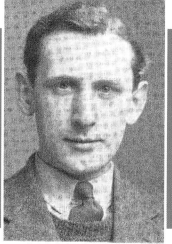

Some student memories of Buccleuch Street in the 1940s

Rod Campbell and Harry Pfaff recall their time at Buccleuch Street in 1941 and 1942.

Rod Campbell graduated in 1946 and lectured and researched in pathology until 1969. He was then appointed Foundation Head of a new Graduate School of Tropical Veterinary Science which later metamorphosed into a full veterinary school at James Cook University in Australia. Harry Pfaff, a 1947 graduate and a famed veterinary practitioner throughout Glasgow was awarded an Honorary Fellowship by the University of Glasgow in 2003 for his work on small animal medicine, vaccination development and the identification of feline leukaemia virus with Bill Jarrett.[74,75]

Rod Campbell could not imagine a place less suitable for a veterinary school than the old Victorian pumping station. 'The nearest farm was twenty miles away.

In their clinical courses, at the time, students saw only the occasional horse, though at the back, the Pathology Department conducted a brisk diagnostic trade with cattle, sheep, pigs, poultry, zoo animals and innumerable cats and dogs that generated a mass of significant research. It is doubtful if the School would receive accreditation today. Yet for a time in its latter years the building was the place of work of a future Nobel Prize-winner, Fellows of the Royal Society and Royal Society of Edinburgh, Directors of Institutes and numerous Professors. Oxbridge it was not, but it produced the goods.

There was a dismal students' common room that hosted Friday night dances of immortal memory and cabarets that would have compared favourably with the Cambridge Footlights. Even the staff held parties there when Ellen Leighton, a German refugee, gourmet chef and pathology technician served exquisite meals and senior lecturers played ventriloquist and dummy or sang lieder by Hugo Wolff. We were a cultured mob. There was no Student Union but a caretaker lady dispensed tea and cheese and tomato rolls for the hungry.'

Harry Pfaff described some of their lecturers. They were taught animal management by George Weir who invented a type of horseshoe which could prevent it being jammed in tram lines. In third year they were taught materia medica by Alexander Thomson.

Cannabis was used as a sedative for horses and was sold by the bale. (When Harry Pfaff started practice he kept sugar coated opium balls in old sweetie jars and they were used to treat diarrhoea.) In fourth year they were taught pathology by the strict disciplinarian Professor John 'Bomber' Emslie, so-called as he would bomb on you if you were found to be lacking knowledge when asked a question. Hugh Begg senior taught parasitology, from the text book – Parasitology by Moennig.

Students gained practical experience or 'seeing practice' at the Dog and Cat Free Clinic in Argyle Street run by Ian Lauder. Harry Pfaff also spent time with Mr Mitchell at Anderston Cross who looked after Barr's Irn Bru horses. At that time there were many draught horses in Glasgow. In 1944 and again in 1945, there was a widespread outbreak of equine flu, infecting hundreds of horses and finishing off the working horse in Glasgow.

In 1945-46, following the death of Donald Campbell, fourth and final year students were mainly taught surgery by an emergency consortium of local practitioners led by William Weipers. Both Pfaff and Campbell were present in 1945 for the talk given by the Nobel Prize winner for Medicine for the discovery and development of penicillin, Sir Alexander Fleming when he was invited by the student's Glasgow Veterinary Association. A future Nobel laureate was also in the audience, James Black, Lecturer in Physiology.

1956

The Chair of Animal Husbandry and Veterinary Preventative Medicine established.

25

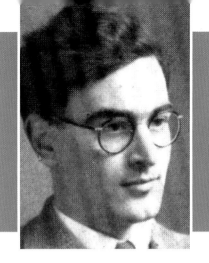

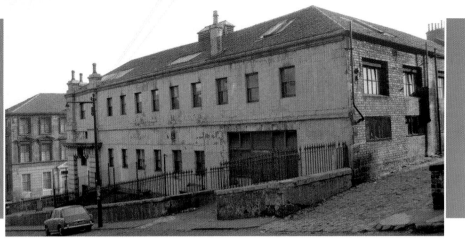

Harry Pfaff

Buccleuch Street 1969

Bill Martin's war time recollections (1942 - 1947)

'We enrolled on leaving school aged seventeen. Most students were male and few came from outside Scotland. During World War II, registration for national service was compulsory at age seventeen and call-up came at eighteen. However students were allowed to defer call-up until their studies were completed, provided they passed their exams. Most of our 1942 class undertook a wartime role such as civil defence, home guard or fire service. Food production was vital, so some veterinary surgeons were called-up for the Royal Veterinary Corp while others were allowed to remain in farm animal practice.' The student's air raid shelter was in the stables where above them, the floor of the main hall had been reinforced with a layer of sandbags.[76]

Transition years, Ken Hosie's recollections from 1945 - 1950

'The first year of the course consisted of chemistry/physics (Dr Joseph Knox), botany/zoology (James 'Seamus' O'Sullivan) who worked single-handed, and anatomy (Helen 'Nellie' Smith) who was later assisted by Flora Lindsay and Finlay McCallum. The teaching of anatomy was continued in the second year and was a detailed study of the horse with comparative consideration of the dog, ox, sheep and pig.

Dissection was carried out on preserved specimens kept in tanks of formaldehyde solution. There being no special provision for students to wash after dissecting, many left the building reeking of formaldehyde.

In second year both physiology/biochemistry and histology (Robert Aitken) were added to gross anatomy, and additional lectures on embryology/developmental anatomy were given by Drs George Wyburn and Paul Bacsich of Glasgow University Anatomy Department. Bob Aitken was assisted in the teaching laboratory by Miss Elspeth Eadie (biochemistry) and Robin Maneely (histology). There was no provision for laboratory work in physiology. During this year a number of ex-servicemen entered the course replacing some of the previous first year entrants from school who had fallen by the wayside at the first professional examinations.

The third year subjects were animal management and materia medica (Alexander Thomson) and nutrition and hygiene (Nicol Nicolson). These did not involve any practical work as it was expected that such would be acquired while seeing practice with general practitioners.

The fourth year was devoted to pathology/bacteriology and parasitology. Lectures on pathology were given by Prof John Emslie and Rod Campbell who also conducted post-mortem examinations and ran the histopathology classes with the assistance of Adolf Watrach.

Bacteriology was taught by Stanislaw Michna assisted by a Mr Nicholas. The course on parasitology was delivered by George Urquhart and Seamus O'Sullivan.

The fifth (final) year subjects were medicine and surgery. Lectures on veterinary medicine were delivered by George Dykes and Carlyle McCance. The only contact with farm animals was by visiting the slaughterhouse and meat market in Bell Street. Some experience of small animal conditions was gained at the PDSA clinic run by Ian Lauder in Argyle Street, but was mostly dependent on seeing small animal practice with private practitioners.

Surgery was taught by the Principal Albert Forsyth but mostly by Donald Lawson, but as in other clinical subjects there was little opportunity to see actual surgery within the college building. Some lectures on meat inspection were given by Sydney Abbot, Nicol Nicolson and Carlyle McCance at the meat market where specimens of disease could be seen.'

In 1949 all this was about to change. The college was finally incorporated into the University of Glasgow. William Weipers, a local veterinary practitioner and Chairman of the Board of Governors of the Veterinary College, with a keen desire to improve veterinary education, was appointed Director of Veterinary Education in the College, henceforth known as the University of Glasgow Veterinary School.

Chapter Three

Veterinary Education in the University Era

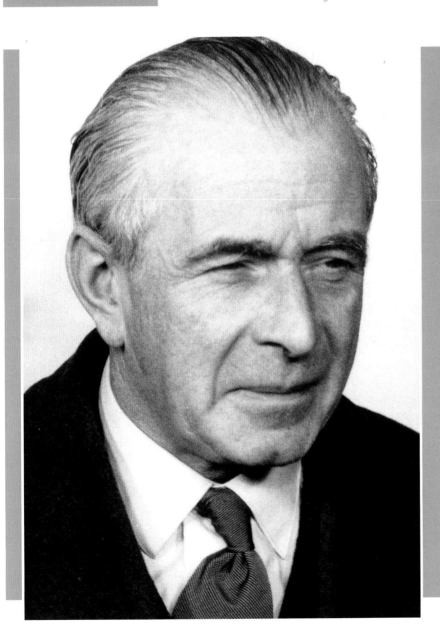

New Director, William Weipers

Following the second Loveday Report, there had been some discussion whether the University of Glasgow would take in the old Veterinary College or start up a new school in opposition.

Over the twentyfive years of his leadership, Sir William established the Glasgow Veterinary School as one of the finest in Europe, gaining worldwide recognition for its teaching and research. It was said that Sir William's greatest asset was his judgement of people and this allowed him to select an outstanding group of young veterinary scientists who developed the research strengths of the school to the level which exists today. He continued to support the School in his retirement when it was threatened with closure following the Riley Report.

Sir William's significant research contributions to veterinary education and research were acknowledged by honorary degrees from Glasgow and Stirling Universities, his election to the Royal Society of Edinburgh and his fellowship and presidency of the Royal College of Veterinary Surgeons 1964-1965. He received a Knighthood in 1966. The Weipers Centre for Equine Welfare (opened in 1995) and the Sir William Weipers Memorial Lecture are named in his honour.[77,78]

Sir William was Head of the School from 1949 to 1974. He retired after twentyfive years with the University of Glasgow, leading the College, School and Faculty.

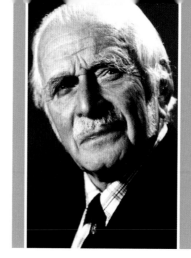

A scientific conference and Silver Jubilee celebration was held to mark his retirement. The programme reflected the many achievements of the Vet School during his twenty five years.[79] There was a wonderful dinner-dance on the final Saturday evening. The whole celebration was held in marquees on the lawn in the Estate by the River Kelvin over a beautiful sunny few days towards the end of June. When the marquees were taken down, it started to rain.

When it was accepted that the College would be part of the University of Glasgow, Sir Hector Hetherington, Principal of the University of Glasgow disagreed with William Weipers, at that time Chairman of the Board of Governors of the Veterinary College, over the degree awarded and the location of the new School. Hetherington would have liked the degree to be in Veterinary Science and be a part of the Science Faculty with pre-clinical classes in Gilmorehill and clinical departments to be built at Auchincruive in the grounds of the Agricultural College. He 'did not wish to hear the sound of cattle lowing on Gilmorehill'.[80] Weipers was anxious that the School should be part of the Faculty of Medicine; he felt that 'we are a science but we are what I call practitioners of medical science. We practise in the same way but in different species from the medicals who practise human medicine but both lean heavily on medical science'.[81]

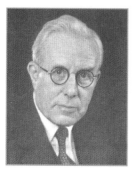

On 1 October 1949, the School was established as a sub-faculty within the Faculty of Medicine of the University of Glasgow under a Board of Veterinary Studies. Forty students enrolled.[82]

Sir Hector Hetherington

The post of Principal disappeared and William Weipers (later Sir William) was appointed as Director of Veterinary Education.[83] Widely regarded as an inspired and visionary appointment, he came to be known as the father of the modern University of Glasgow Veterinary School.[84]

William Weipers, a son of the manse, had a long association with the Glasgow Veterinary College. Born in Kilbirnie, Ayrshire, he was the son of the Church of Scotland parish minister. His mother came from a farming community in Aberdeenshire. The family moved to Glasgow and he was educated at Whitehill Higher Grade School in Dennistoun, but considered himself a late developer. His primary interest was farming and after spending eighteen months with a Kirkcudbright livestock farmer, he enrolled at the Glasgow Veterinary College in 1920 for the four year course.

Though he thought it described best by Sir Hector Hetherington as the 'first rate second class academic slum of Europe', he enjoyed the educational set up.[85] He received first class certificates in biology, chemistry, stable management, higher anatomy, hygiene, medicine, surgery, and silver medals in anatomy, physiology, pathology and materia medica.[86] He won a prize in every class he took. In second year he was taught anatomy by Professor Whitehouse (later Principal).

In his final year, he worked with a local practitioner, David Imrie. Weipers combined early morning work, academia and surgeries when he was left in charge of Imrie's practice. He remembered his first case, a horse breathing very quickly in one of the stables in Govan which was quickly diagnosed as having tetanus by Imrie. Diagnosis then was based on observation and ancillary aids were rarely used.

Weipers then studied for a year in Edinburgh and took his Diploma in Veterinary Medicine. This allowed him to gain experience in aseptic surgery with Professor Mitchell who had taken a medical qualification and returned to the Edinburgh College to apply new techniques from human surgery. Weipers took a clinical assistant's post for £3 per week and stayed in Edinburgh for two and a half years, despite being a 'Glasgow man'.

He started his practice in the West End of Glasgow in 1929 and was inundated with surgical work when word got around that he could do abdominal surgery and the animal would recover! Many students from the Veterinary College saw practice with him. He was also one of the few vets to own his own X-ray machine.

1957

Glasgow develops the use of tissue culture for the diagnosis of canine distemper.

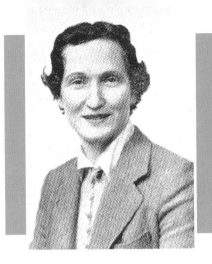

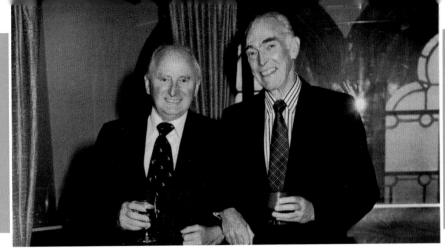

Weipers continued to learn from medical specialists including 'Pa Hutton' who was the surgeon in the Western Infirmary, John Marshall in the Eye Infirmary and Eddie Connel, an ear, nose and throat specialist. He also became known as a bit of an expert on wallabies: Lady Forteviot had brought some over from Australia and they had developed canker and necrosis of the tail from running through the ice and slush.

Weipers married Mary McLean, from Barra in 1939 and formed a lifelong association with the Island. Mary later studied at the Veterinary College in Buccleuch Street and graduated in 1952.[87,88] At the time that Weipers became Director, she managed the small hospital and kennels which he had built at Duntocher.[89]

William Weipers had two key supporters, his senior administrator John Roberts and his secretary, Betty Gordon. Following National Service as a navigator in the Royal Air Force and a stint with a local authority, John Roberts, affectionately known as 'JR' joined the University of Glasgow in 1957 as an administrative assistant to Weipers.

Roberts was responsible for the day to day running of the newly built Veterinary Hospital at Garscube. In the early days there, life was dominated by the Tannoy public address system which regularly announced 'telephone for Mr Roberts', amusing the students and annoying the local residents in Ilay Road.

During this time, there was a lot of building work and he was in the thick of it. In 1968, when Faculty status was established, he became the first Clerk to the Faculty of Veterinary Medicine and held the post until he retired in 1989.

He had been involved in the considerable work required in the establishment of the new Faculty. He worked with six Deans and was awarded an honorary MA, a rare award, by Senate in recognition of his services.[90,91]

Betty Gordon was William Weipers's wonderful indefatigable Secretary from 1950 until 1971 at Garscube. She was totally organised and warmly pleasant to all.

In 1971, Betty Blake, following Betty Gordon, joined the staff of the Faculty as secretary to the Dean. She worked there until her retirement in 1995 having been secretary to seven successive Deans. She is remembered by Norman Wright, her final Dean (1991-1999), as a special person to him and to her colleagues and a one off with a prodigious knowledge of the school and staff.[92]

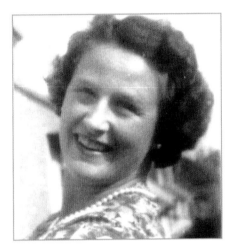

Betty Gordon

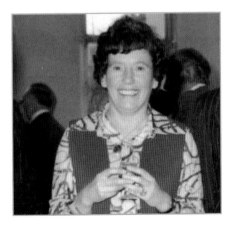

Betty Blake

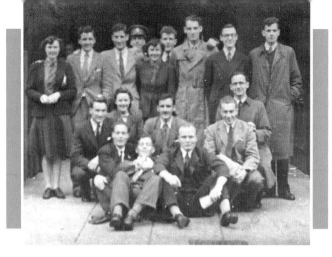

Students 1940s

Student days: work hard play hard

The students of the Glasgow Veterinary School have always had a strong *esprit de corps* built around closely shared experiences of learning and extramural activities. Their ethos was, and remains, 'work hard-play hard'. While gaining their final qualification has been their goal, they never forget to enjoy the journey through the course which is punctuated with social events. Along the way enduring friendships are forged and key academic figures and support staff influence students, sculpting their personalities and paving the pathway for their future.

From 1945 to 1949, conditions at Buccleuch Street had improved slightly with the re-establishment of the grant from the Department of Agriculture. However changes began to accelerate after the merger with the University in 1949. One change was the awarding of degrees; all students who enrolled from October 1949 onwards and who successfully completed the course received a Glasgow University degree of Bachelor of Veterinary Medicine and Surgery (BVMS) which allowed membership of the RCVS.

Jimmy Armour's student days 1947-52

This period coincided with a marked change in the composition of the student body due to the influx of servicemen returning from World War II. The demands placed on the lecturing staff increased as these more mature students pressed for information on the latest knowledge. This proved difficult for some of the staff who were local practitioners working on a part-time basis. The supply of clinical material was particularly poor and experience gained when seeing practice was a key element in clinical training. Fortunately this situation improved dramatically with the appointments of outstanding clinicians such as Weipers, McIntyre, Lawson, Martin and Lauder once the University took over and the new facilities opened at Garscube.

The post war phase also witnessed an uplift in social activities and the Friday night dances at Buccleuch Street became the place to be for Glasgow's student population. Music was provided from a variety of sources and often included Bill Jarrett (trumpet) and Bill Horn (clarinet).

The 'Dick Days' at which a range of sports were contested were special with Glasgow dominating in soccer and the Dick Boys shining at rugby. The evenings were riotous affairs and many incidents do not bear reprinting. One amusing altercation occurred when one Glasgow student with familial knowledge of train engines, his father and uncle both being train drivers, started the Waverley to Glasgow last train of the day and moved it a few yards until the security guard descended on him. The story grew and it became part of folklore that he drove it all the way to Glasgow. Ian Smith, the student involved, later became a Professor at the RVC in London.

The annual trip 'Doon the Watter (Clyde)' every June was another popular event, although the crew of MacBraynes' steamer involved took a long time to recover.

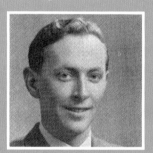

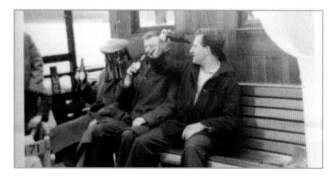

'Doon the Watter'

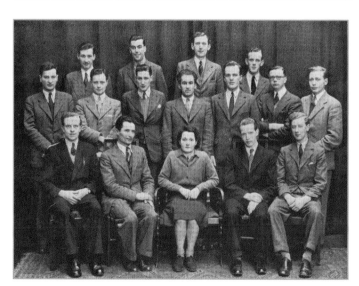

Staff 1946

1961
Chair of Veterinary Medicine established.

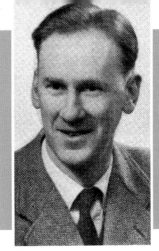
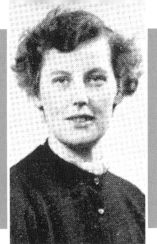

Among those returning from military service after World War II there was a plethora of real characters, one of whom, Matt Cunningham became a member of staff in the 1950s. Before pursuing a career in East Africa, Matt joined the Fleet Air Arm in the early 1940s, and after training in Canada qualified as a pilot officer. Following service on various fronts he was demobbed in 1946 and entered the vet course at Glasgow in December 1947 joining at the end of the first term, as did many of his fellow ex servicemen.

He was an excellent student who never seemed to do a lot of studying and participated in all social and sporting events.

He joined the Medicine Department as a large animal house surgeon in 1953, became an (assistant) lecturer working on Johne's disease and Mucosal Disease until 1958. Matt was a larger than life character, afraid of nothing or no one, a top class mountaineer and deep sea fisherman, never without a packet of cigarettes, once encountered, never forgotten.

The University also began to create professorial chairs in veterinary subjects. William Weipers was awarded the first chair in Veterinary Surgery and John Emslie the chair of Veterinary Pathology. Others followed with five professorial chairs established between 1951 and 1963.

Veterinary Surgery 1951 William Weipers
Veterinary Pathology 1951 John Emslie
Animal Husbandry and Veterinary Preventive Medicine 1956 Scott Inglis
Veterinary Medicine 1961 Ian McIntyre
Veterinary Physiology 1963 Bill Mulligan[93,94]

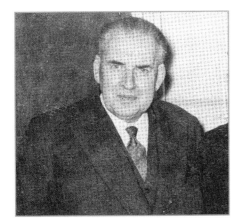

John Emslie

Staff, old and new

In 1950 the number of staff was relatively small (twenty) but as the school moved into its next phase William Weipers had the opportunity to recruit new staff from veterinary, medical and scientific backgrounds facilitating both outstanding teaching and research.
By 1960 the number of academic staff had more than doubled to fortyfour and similar increases occurred in the numbers of support staff. Twenty years later by 1980 academic staff numbers had risen to nearly seventy.

Although staff numbers in 1950 were limited, many of these academics would have long-lasting influences on the Veterinary School and its students. In addition to Weipers and Emslie the staff roll included Helen (Nellie) Smith, Flora Lindsay and Findlay McCallum (veterinary anatomy); Bob (Joe) Aitken (veterinary histology); Alexander Thomson (animal management); Ian Lauder and Bill Martin (small animal clinic), George Dykes and Carlyle McCance (veterinary medicine); George Urquhart, Rod Campbell, Seamus O'Sullivan and Stanislaw Michna (veterinary pathology); Donald Lawson (veterinary surgery) and Jimmy Black (veterinary physiology,).

During the 1950s the staff membership expanded to include new key individuals such as Scott Inglis and Gordon Hemingway (animal husbandry); Bill Mulligan, Frank Jennings, Tom Douglas and Ian Aitken (veterinary biochemistry); Ian McIntyre, Alastair Greig, Ted Fisher, Rodger Dalton, (veterinary medicine); Angus Dunn and Jimmy Armour (veterinary parasitology), Hugh McCusker and John Hamilton (veterinary pathology); Bill Jarrett, Craig Sharp and Hugh Pirie (hospital pathology); John Sanford (veterinary pharmacology); Eric Pickering, Ronald Anderson and David Robertshaw (veterinary physiology); Sidney Jennings, Jimmy Campbell and Peter Hignett (veterinary surgery).

Leading members of the support staff recruited in the 1950s who played a key role in the School throughout their careers included Ian Maclean (veterinary biochemistry and later physiology), Ken Bairden (the senior technician in veterinary parasitology). Charlie Keanie drove the van which transported samples between Garscube and Buccleuch Street every day, Eddie Quinn who ran the animal house, Pat Hanlon in the main office who paid out the weekly wages and Mrs Taylor who managed the canteen. Weipers appreciated fully the significance of using equipment of the highest quality. This included the importance of pictorial presentation for teaching, research and for conference presentation. Thus, Archie Finnie, a professional photographer, was employed from the 1950s, to be joined in the 1970s by Alan May. The quality of their work was unsurpassed and Glasgow had a world class reputation not only for its research and teaching, but also for the excellence and innovation of its pictorial presentations.

Memories of the 1950s from George Barr, a renowned Ayrshire Practitioner

I phoned the vet school in 1950, at the age of seventeen, seeking entrance, had a Saturday interview with Prof Weipers in Buccleuch Street at which he asked what farming experience I had (worked on a local farm from age eleven) and was promised a place after completing six Highers which I managed. I was in the second year of the BVMS course which had started in 1949. The course started at Anderson College for the First year with botany, zoology, physics and chemistry. A poor timetable gave the forty students three free afternoons a week in the first term. The botany lecturer encouraged us to buy a book of no value to us, but which had his name as co-author. The physics lecturer, poor man, had a squeaky voice and lectured with difficulty. We had all the dental students in for this subject and he was teased mercilessly. It was the only exam I failed first time. Chemistry was taken by Dr Chisholm, a very precise gentleman and his subject was mostly reckoned to be the hardest but most useful. The dull first year was only enlightened by the excitement of a lecture on animal management from a Glasgow practitioner, Alex Thomson which was our first real connection with veterinary work.

I should say that we were a very mixed bunch. Quite a few of the class had done National Service and were a bit older and more mature, and we had a Polish student in his 30s and three girls, plus a few of the previous year who had fallen back. When at the old College we met up with some much older MRCVS students, some who had struggled for years. World War II had ended just five years before I started and there was still some food rationing.

We really got into it in Second Year. The College at Buccleuch Street was very primitive, no doubt established when the horse was king. We had anatomy on the ground floor with Mrs Smith and Flora MacDonald, both very capable, but known to have sent the odd student to sleep.

Joe Aitken gave us histology and embryology with much writing. Physiology was from Dr James Black, whose intense interest in research meant he usually appeared twenty to thirty minutes late for the lecture, which was always enthusiastically given. Dr Mulligan, a lovely man, did biochemistry.

While we were aware that something was happening at Garscube, we didn't get there till Third Year for materia medica, taken in a hay loft with bales. It was a very outdated subject, with antibiotics hardly mentioned, but we learned about a mel (a drug in honey). Prof Scott Inglis gave us animal husbandry. At least we felt we were getting on our way. Back at College, we had the 'Bomber'- (Prof Emslie) for pathology and Dr Michna for bacteriology. The 'Bomber' was notorious for bearing down hard on students and having girls in tears. Things were made lighter in the common room where snacks were served and table tennis was greatly enjoyed on a table which dipped at each end. Parasitology was presented by Seamus O'Sullivan, a dapper and precise man.

In Fourth and Final Years the course became much more integrated, though the Medicine and Surgery departments were often at loggerheads. We were fortunate to have research workers as lecturers. The team responsible for lungworm vaccination was there, with Prof Jarrett et al. We also were fortunate to have as lecturers Drs. Ian McIntyre, Bill Martin and Ian Lauder. Prof Donald Lawson did small animal surgery in a loosebox with stable doors and Mr Sydney Jennings did large animal surgery, mostly outside. Although much was primitive we had the advantage of seeing constant improvements in the facilities. Only fourteen of the original forty of us who started in 1950 finished in July 1955, though others joined us who had failed previous years.

Most of the time I enjoyed GUVS and am a proud graduate!

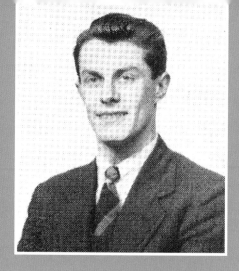

Student admissions

In order to gain entry to the veterinary course applicants had to achieve a 'Certificate of Fitness' which specified they had attained the minimum entry requirements including grades in the necessary subjects – a language other than English remained a requirement until the 1980s! In addition, interviews were held at the main University, usually in the Robing Room, and conditional offers would be made to the lucky applicants. In the 1960s each intake included a handful of women, usually five, plus a number of overseas students who usually were from African countries which did not have their own veterinary schools.

New curriculum

Following the merger with the University and a revision of the curriculum, four basic science subjects were taught in the First Year by University departments at Gilmorehill, namely chemistry, physics, botany and zoology while other veterinary subjects such as anatomy (including embryology), physiology, biochemistry and histology continued to be taught at the old site in Buccleuch Street. Clinical teaching began to take place at Garscube following the construction of the Veterinary Hospital building in the early 1950s.

1962
Chair of Veterinary Physiology established.

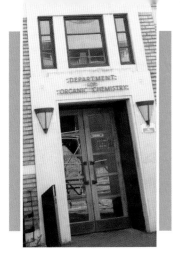

Chemistry Building Gilmorehill

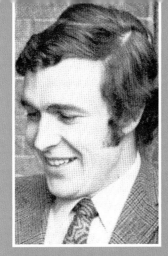

Students therefore moved between Gilmorehill, Buccleuch Street and Garscube for their classes and became integrated with the student body at Gilmorehill, at least during the early part of the course.

The basic science subjects taught at Gilmorehill were not popular with students. However a strict 'class ticket' system operated whereby students had to gain at least 35 percent in the term exams to be allowed to enter the professional examinations. In the case of physics and chemistry the First Professional Examination took place after only two terms at Easter and a failure in that exam could delay entry into the Second Year and possible exclusion from the course if the subject was subsequently failed at the resits. The physics and chemistry lectures were given jointly to students of veterinary medicine, human medicine and dentistry resulting in more than 300 students being present. Many of the students, especially the English, had already studied these subjects to quite an advanced level at school. These factors combined with the tendency for the lectures to be delivered by junior members of staff created a situation in which it was very difficult to keep order in the lectures and mayhem frequently ensued.

Traditionally the five year curriculum was strictly divided into pre-clinical, (Years 1 and 2) para-clinical (Year 3) and clinical years (Years 4 and 5) so that students had to wait until the Fourth Year before any significant clinical training was provided. Each subject boundary was usually jealously guarded by its department. The Head of Department was usually a long term appointment and held considerable power and influence.

Although the First Year was dominated by physics, chemistry, botany and zoology there was some exposure to veterinary anatomy. This was a major course extending over five terms and involved over 400 hours of instruction. For the whole of the Second Year of the course students spent half of every day in the anatomy laboratory. This began with a roll call of the students and a lecture followed by several hours in the dissection laboratory.

Extensive dissections were carried out on specimens which were preserved in formalin and the smell could be over-powering. These sessions were also accompanied by extensive discourse on politics, football and the other sex.

By the Third Year 'diseases' entered the vocabulary and there were intensive courses in pathology, parasitology and microbiology occupying four terms. The first lecture of the Pathology course was traditionally given by Professor Emslie on the subject of inflammation. In parasitology and microbiology most of the teaching was based on systematic learning of parasite life cycles and the culturing and diagnostic features of the families of bacteria. Virology was taught in a relatively small number of lectures. There were brief introductions to veterinary medicine, surgery and obstetrics. Veterinary materia medica, pharmacy and pharmacology occupied two terms.

In the Fourth Year instruction in veterinary medicine, veterinary surgery and reproduction began. A highlight (and a major strength of the Glasgow course) was the integration of clinical medicine with pathology. Post mortem demonstrations were held on an almost daily basis at lunchtime and featured many of the cases which the students had examined as clinical cases. Many of the senior staff of the Medicine and Hospital Pathology departments were present at these demonstrations. These sessions became the stuff of legends with vigorous discussions often ensuing. Other consequences were the stimulation of research programmes, publications and student motivation to follow an academic career.

The Final Year was dominated by weekly clinical rotations through the four departments of large animal medicine, small animal medicine, veterinary surgery and reproduction. Lectures continued to be held throughout the Final Year and these were frequently augmented by outside speakers.

Jimmy Murphy, from the start in the 1950s, with the able assistance of Richard Irvine, was the Emperor of the Post-Mortem Room. His rule lasted over forty years. He was a remarkable, tough, hardworking, charismatic character who ran a spotlessly efficient operation on behalf of Bill Jarrett. His powers of observation were unsurpassed, as he prepared the huge number of necropsies that passed through his hands. These were from the major research programmes in parasitology, virology and cancer,

as well as the clinical cases that came through the small animal and equine hospitals, and the farm animals purchased for clinical teaching purposes, and followed by the students to PM demonstrations. The stream of students and young pathologists who trained under Jimmy received a remarkable experience. Jimmy was also a fully qualified meat inspector and was responsible for the certified abattoir at Garscube. There were many favoured members of staff who were able to delight in the experience of well butchered well hung meat.

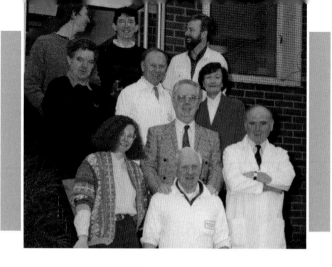

Jimmy Murphy (front) outside PM room

Practical experience off-site

Although most of the formal education of veterinary students took place at the veterinary school, there was essential off-site training, the most important of which was 'seeing practice'. A total of twentysix weeks of experience was required to be undertaken (and still is) by each student during the vacations from the beginning of Second Year (students now start extramural studies in First Year). Most of this was undertaken in private practice but up to four weeks laboratory work could also be included. Students were encouraged to seek a range of experience across large and small animal practice and were expected to keep a case book as this formed part of the Final Examination. Students frequently failed to keep up to date with their case books and as the Finals approached there was discrete exchanging of 'cases' between students.

In addition to the major task of 'seeing practice' there was other off-site training. Meat inspection techniques were overseen by Lyle McCance at the Meat Market in Duke Street, a huge old-style slaughterhouse complex which seemed to be populated by a special tribe of knife-brandishing Glaswegians. An equally disturbing experience, also supervised by Lyle McCance, was when classes of students were taken to large dairy farms attached to the Victorian mental hospitals on the outskirts of Glasgow to practice rectal palpation and the examination of the feet of cattle. The hospital inmates would frequently be in attendance and caused alarm. For many years it was a requirement that every veterinary student learnt to ride and in the 1960s classes were held at Kilmardinny. The horses and the students were equally unenthusiastic but fortunately the final test of riding ability was very unchallenging. Another tradition in the 1960s was the lambing course whereby students learnt lambing skills prior to being turned loose on sheep farms at Easter in the Second and Third Years of the course. Instruction was under the watchful eye of Peter Hignett and Jean Renton. Training was provided using dead lambs placed in various contortions within a plastic bag (artificial uterus) in the pelvic skeleton of a sheep. Students also honed their lambing skills on the Cochno flock and at the Home Farm and this involved rotas of students giving twentyfour hour cover.

Sporting vets

Given the relatively low numbers of veterinary students and graduates at Glasgow University compared with other subject areas, the contribution by the vets to sporting success has been remarkable.

Pride of place has to go to our Olympians namely Angus Carmichael who played in the British Soccer Team in the 1948 Olympics in London and reached the semi-final and David Gracie who represented Britain in the 440 Hurdles at the 1952 Helsinki Games and was the fastest losing semi-finalist in an era when only six reached the final.

At Commonwealth Games level, Quintin McKellar represented Scotland in rowing in 1986 and Hayley Haining in athletics in 1998. (Quintin also succeeded Jimmy Armour as Staff President of the University Athletic Cub). David Logue represented Northern Ireland in the marathon. Alan Wilson (BVMS 1986) ran for Great Britain in the Marathon and Scotland on track and cross country between 1983-1987.

At international level, Scotland Caps were awarded for soccer to Billy Steel (B cap) and David Seawright (amateur) while in rugby Euan Murray amassed many caps and toured South Africa with the British and Irish Lions. A plethora of University Blues were awarded to vet students in a wide range of sports including athletics, soccer, golf, hockey, rugby, shinty, squash and swimming. In many instances those obtaining blues represented Scottish Universities and also played at district level.

Of those who became members of staff special mention should be made of Craig Sharp who apart from his own sporting achievements in athletics and squash became a famous sports physiologist and was adviser to several British Olympic Teams. Jim Bogan was an outstanding long distance runner and took part in several national and international events. Jimmy Armour was the British Boys Golf Champion, Hoylake, in 1947 and then later as a Third Year student qualified in the 1950 Open Championship. Along with Tom Douglas he also qualified to compete in the National Golf Championship in the early 50s.

Undergraduate research training

This programme was born out of the PM demonstrations. During these sessions recent research work on-going in the school and occasionally in East Africa were often discussed. These stimulated several undergraduates to enquire about the possibility of vacational work in research laboratories. This programme started in earnest in the 1960s until by the 1990s had developed into a formal summer school which attracted about a quarter of the students. During the summer of 2011 there were about thirty undergraduates, mostly between their Third and Fourth Year of study undertaking summer projects of between six and eight weeks duration. They may be funded externally through, for instance, Biotechnology and Biological Sciences Research Council (BBSRC) or The Wellcome Trust, or internally by the School. Research areas range from basic lab-based science, sometimes in collaboration with the Moredun Research Institute, through to more clinically orientated projects. In addition, students are involved in data acquisition and analysis related to animal welfare and epidemiology and in the provision of new educational materials. Many students elect to present their project results to peers at the Governors' and Mitchell of Cranstonhill Prize competition, and some present results at scientific meetings and through published articles. Over the years many of these students who participated have travelled to the top of the profession worldwide in academic research, commerce, and general practice.

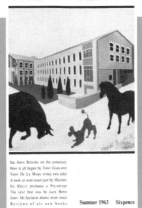

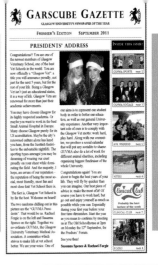

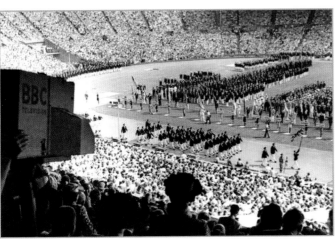

1948 Olympics in London

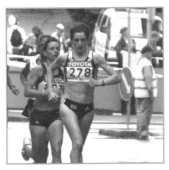

Hayley Haining

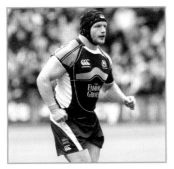

Euan Murray

Freshers Social and the Garscube Gazette

Another important and longstanding tradition was the Freshers Social at which the First Year students were entertained by students from the other Years. The key feature was a review in which there was much lampooning of the staff. Considerable talent was displayed by the students in the lyrics, music and acting. William Weipers and senior members of staff sat along the front row and took it all in good heart. In the 1960s key performers included Sandy Weipers (impersonating his uncle William), Alan Shearer and Colin Silver's rendition of 'Wee Johnnie's Lost His Jaurie' (which is a Scots word for marble), and Jimmy Duncan and Jack Boyd with their famous song 'The Scottish Tomcat' to the tune of Andy Stewart's 'The Scottish Soldier'. The students produced an annual magazine, The Veteran, which was the organ of report for all the social and sporting news and an opportunity for budding features writers. Its functions were taken over by the Garscube Gazette. With the campus split between Buccleuch Street, Gilmorehill and Garscube, students founded the Gazette in November 1962, which was intended to lay new lines of communication and supply information about the College and student activities and to bridge the gap between staff and students and the early and later Years of the College. It provided news, a letters page, surveys, advice and events as well as reviews of the Fresher's Social and annual concert and dance, all for tuppence. The first editor-in-chief was Hugh B. Lewis, helped out by assistant editors from each year. Ian Sloan took over in 1965. He remembers that 'Isobel Cairns, a secretary at Garscube, typed out all the Roneo sheets for us. No photocopying or computers in those days.'

The last Freshers Social to be held in Buccleuch Street took place in 1968. The talking point was the high number of females, 'eighteen girls out of a class of fortytwo'. By 1969, most students had moved into the new building and 'Buccleuch Street is being let to the Geophysics Department... with pleasure'[95] The Freshers' Socials continue and The Gazette is produced annually, principally to give the Freshers an introduction to the students' Glasgow University Veterinary Medical Association and what to expect in the first year of study.

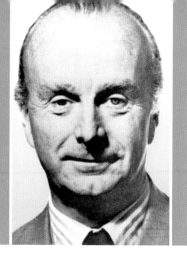

In 1974 Ian McIntyre became the Dean of the recently established Faculty of Veterinary Medicine and as such played a notable role in the Council of the RCVS, where he served among others on the Education Committee until 1980, and was Chairman from 1976 – 1980; the Parliamentary Committee; and the Specialisation and Further Education Committee.

Ian McIntyre the second Dean (1974 - 1977)

Friday night dances

An important tradition at the Veterinary College in Buccleuch Street stretching back for many decades and lasting until the School left the site in 1969 was the Friday night dances in the common room of the College. These were organised by the students and became famous, or more correctly, infamous. They were a key social event of the week at which vet students, 90 percent of whom were male, had the opportunity to meet girls, mostly from other colleges. Those from the Domestic Science College (the 'Dough' school) were particularly popular and judged to eventually make good wives, as well as ladies from the Glasgow School of Art just round the corner in Renfrew Street, though perhaps not considered in the same way!

The dances were organised for and by the vet students but they were frequently gatecrashed and within reason a blind eye was given to this because it created extra revenue for the students. Security at the main door and the selling of tickets was a key job and allocated to veterinary students on a rota. Security at the Friday night dances was discretely overseen by Jimmy Brooks, the avuncular Janitor who during the normal working day wore a splendid uniform or a more practical brown overall. He knew almost everything that went on in the School including all the gossip from these dances. The income generated by the dances was considerable and supported many of the activities that became part of the student social year including the Vet Ball, the Final Year Dinner and Year Book, Dick Day, the Vet Cruise and the Rodeo.

Vet School Centenary 1962

In 1962, the Veterinary School celebrated one hundred years since its foundation (and thirteen years with the Faculty of Medicine). To mark the centenary, a programme of events was arranged which included scientific demonstrations and a reception by the Court of the University at the Veterinary Hospital at Garscube, followed by a dinner-dance at the North British Station Hotel (now the Millennium Hotel next to Queen Street Station on George Square). The centenary fund was established to provide student amenities at Garscube and Cochno. [96] Students held their own centenary party in Buccleuch Street. [97] In Sir William's address, he reflected that the Glasgow Veterinary College spanned less than a fifth of the life of the University. However, he concluded that 'a hundred years is a long time and a complete scientific revolution has taken place. The impact on the veterinary profession has been great'. He added that 'we have made a beginning'. He paid tribute to Sir Hector Hetherington for his help in establishing the 'enfant terrible' which was the Vet School in the early days. 'The terrible component may have survived as a vestige but there is no doubt that the juvenile phase has passed'. A full account can be found in the Veterinary Record, 1963. [98]

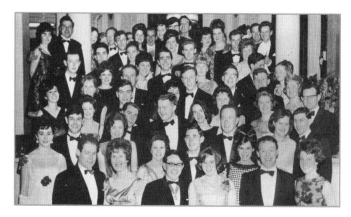

Vet Ball 1964

The Veterinary School becomes the Faculty of Veterinary Medicine 1968

The School grew in significance, and became independent from the Faculty of Medicine in 1968 when the Faculty of Veterinary Medicine was established and William Weipers was appointed the first Dean. The Department of Pathology moved to Garscube in 1968, followed by the Department of Veterinary Anatomy in 1969 when Buccleuch Street closed its doors for the last time. [99]

New professors - real and titular

Starting in the 1970s the number of professors began to increase significantly through the creation of new Chairs and through the promotion of staff to a new category of 'Titular Professor'. This was an innovative and successful development by the University of Glasgow in order to retain and recognise key members of staff. The latter carried the title 'Professor' but lacked the status and salary of the 'real' professors; 'real' Professors had automatically become the head of their respective Department until they retired or moved on. All vacant Chairs were filled following international advertisement and interview. In the 1990s the distinction between Real and Titular Professors faded rapidly and persons appointed to recognised University Chairs no longer necessarily headed their Department.

1963
The first official Faculty link with Africa involving undergraduate education in Kenya is formed.

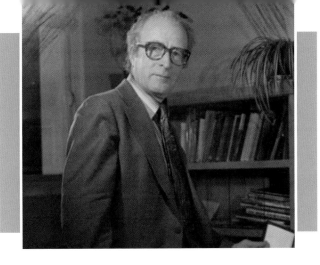

Bill Mulligan served as Dean of the Faculty for three years. It was a period of relative calm before the stringent cuts to University funding which came in the early 1980s when Bill had moved to the role of Vice-Principal for Science.

'The incorporation of the Glasgow Veterinary School into the university system brought about profound and rapid changes in the activity of the School.

This was most far reaching in the increased emphasis on research.

The recruitment of new members of staff, some already established in research, and the encouragement and support of the Director, William Weipers, provided the right environment for research to flourish.'
Professor Bill Mulligan

Bill Mulligan the third Dean (1977 - 1980)

Purchase of the Lanark Practice

The Veterinary School sought to widen the scope of undergraduate clinical teaching through the purchase of a Lanarkshire veterinary practice owned by Mr Douglas Steele in 1978. The University of Glasgow bought it through a combination of a bank loan and royalties from the Dictol vaccine. It was predominantly a farm animal practice, serving farms within a twenty-mile radius of Lanark and employed four veterinary surgeons. Following design and building of new premises, the students from the Veterinary School arrived in October 1981. Robert Plenderleith became the first head of the practice followed by David Anderson.

The practice was well equipped with modern facilities for anaesthesia, radiography, ultrasonic scanning, all types of surgery and intensive animal care. A practice laboratory performed all routine bacteriology and parasitology, while the 'Vet Test 8008' biochemistry analyser developed at the School could process blood samples quickly. All client records were computerised and clinical details were accessible. The facilities were a tremendous asset for both clinical diagnosis and student teaching. An adjoining wing provided accommodation for students and allowed them to participate fully in all aspects of the practice including emergency out-of-hours call outs.[100] The Lanark Practice was eventually sold.

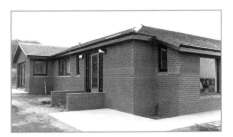

Lanark Practice

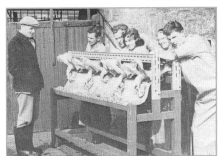

Obstetrics 1960s

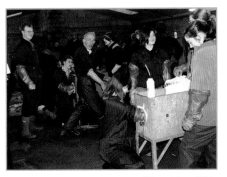

Obstetrics 1990s

A lecture-free final year

Ian McIntyre, with the backing of William Weipers, revolutionised the clinical teaching programme. He established links with vets throughout Scotland and beyond to attract clinical cases which would provide final year students with the skills needed for clinical practice. He also developed the concept of a lecture-free final year in which the students would rotate through a range of clinical stations, spending time with individual cases and debate these in small groups with clinical staff. While proposed in the late 1960s, it took until the late 1970s for all colleagues to accept this as the way forward. Following much debate, the details of the new Fourth and Final Year curriculum were finally agreed in 1980 and put in place in 1981. The first of the students to have a lecture-free final year graduated in 1982. This required an equally comprehensive reorganisation of the fourth year teaching. This new course was divided into species blocks and many classes were delivered by a multidisciplinary mix of lecturers. Printed notes covering most of the course, essentially amounting to new textbooks, were provided for the students (and eagerly sought by students from other veterinary schools). A key feature was the retention of the post-mortem demonstrations which continued to be held on an almost daily basis. The model of the lecture-free final year has been adopted by all the veterinary schools in the UK and many worldwide, underlining the foresight and vision of the School.

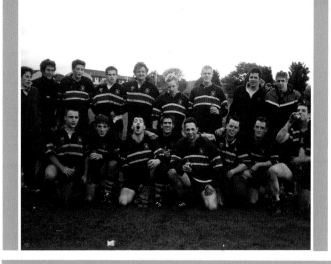

'Hope for the better but prepare for the worst'

During the time of Donald Lawson's Deanship the country was going through a recession. In the University of Glasgow Newsletter, January 1981, Principal Alwyn Williams stated 'our estimates for this academic session are founded on more uncertainties than ever before… There is, of course, always the remote possibility that the government will relent when the full consequence of its policies are understood. But relief, if it comes, is unlikely to be more than marginal. After all, we have already endured five major changes during the last four years, all but one leaving us more impoverished than before in the average unit of resource per student. We have at least learnt to hope for the better while preparing for the worst'.

To address funding issues, discussions within the Faculty in 1981 centred on the possibility of taking in more overseas students at undergraduate and postgraduate level. As the school was equipped to deal with an annual intake of sixty students, this number was maintained for home based students with up to a further five overseas students being admitted.

It was also thought that a taught one year 'Master of Veterinary Medicine' course, comprising a number of electives from various veterinary disciplines, might be attractive and useful to students from developing countries. The Faculty also obtained Senate approval for a new honorary degree of Doctor of Veterinary Medicine and Surgery.[101] Sir William Weipers was the first to receive this honour in 1982.[102]

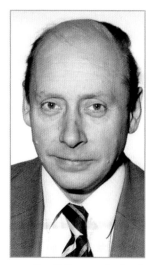

Donald Lawson the fourth Dean (1980 -1983)

1980s Some things change; some things don't

Dom Mellor, BVMS 1991 and Large Animal Clinical Sciences and Public Health Professor of Epidemiology comments.

Some things change:
Class sizes were much smaller then; we were sixty or so in our year, which meant two to a table in dissection, a microscope each and groups of two in the clinics in final year…and the staff still had long summers of student-free time to prepare teaching for the next academic year and do research.

Pie beans and chips, perhaps a bridie if you were lucky, with or without gravy, were pretty much the limits of the culinary delights on offer at lunch time. Salad and fruit were rarely seen, and still more rarely consumed, and there were none of the sophisticated coffee machines we enjoy today.

The 'bear pit' of the old large animal demonstration theatre (sadly now refurbished into an animal-free and specimen-free zone) was compelling attendance for more or less the whole school staff as well as the students in Fourth and Final year. We went there to witness, and learn from, the fierce debates, discussions and just the odd disagreement among an exalted cast of protagonists, prominent among whom were Gibbs, McCandlish, Taylor, Squires, Love, Selman, Thompson, Dalgleish and Pirie.

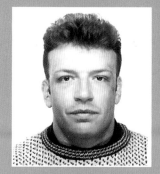

The old GUVMA Hut, decidedly grim by light of day, but decidedly appealing when a combination of alcohol and darkness made it all but invisible during the all-night, ribald, bawdy 'Hut' parties that were such an important component of the Glasgow joie de vivre. The much-vaunted Glasgow 'lecture-free final year' was, for some, only the fifth (or more) and final (perhaps) lecture-free (or virtually so) year of the vet course. Many of those 'correspondence students' passed their exams each year with no problem and have gone on to become and remain very successful members of the Profession.

Some things don't:
The Glasgow student 'esprit de corps' was, and still is, one of the most striking and singular things about the School. The sheer ingenuity and audacity of Glasgow students in their constant pursuit of entertainment, for themselves, their tutors and others, makes the School a very special club of which to be a part. Then, as now, close and informal understanding and trust between staff and students was at the core of this uniquely Glasgow magic. There was a genuine sense of everyone enjoying getting through the course together and, rather like Glasgow itself, whatever was achieved was best achieved with as much humour as possible. The big social events of our calendar in those days were Dick Day, AVS weekend, the Vet Ball, the Half-way Dinner, The Final Year Dinner…just as they remain today. It was, and remains, tremendously exciting to be among so many bright, exuberant and resourceful people.

1964
Feline leukaemia virus first identified by Bill Jarrett.

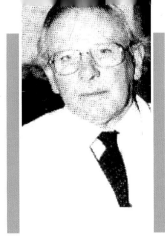

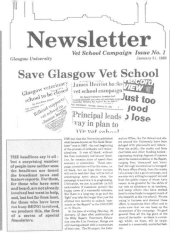

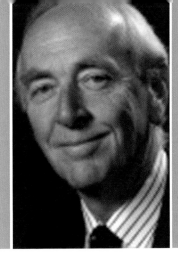

Jimmy Armour became Vice-Principal of the University in 1991. He received a CBE in 1989 and a knighthood in 1995. James Armour reflected 'while the report by Riley and his cohorts dominated my period as Dean, the media exposure and meetings with senior politicians including Prime Minister Thatcher, helped to move the school forward and our relationships with Gilmorehill were never better than post–Riley.' [103]

Tom Douglas, the fifth Dean (1983 -1986)

Jimmy Armour, the sixth Dean (1986 -1991)

History repeats itself - the Riley Report

Shortly after James Armour became Dean in 1986, it was announced that the University Grants Committee (UGC) was considering discontinuing the funding of two veterinary schools in Scotland. Glasgow and Edinburgh were encouraged to discuss how the situation could be resolved. Meetings between the two Principals, Sir Alwyn Williams[104] and Sir John Burnett, and the two Deans Professors James Armour and Ainsley Iggo, from their respective universities and veterinary schools followed. It was proposed that teaching at each school would be merged, with some years held in Glasgow and some in Edinburgh. The Faculty reluctantly agreed. However in 1987, it was announced that the UGC was setting up a Working Party to review veterinary education under the Chairmanship of Sir Ralph Riley with a view to possibly rationalising its provision in the UK.

Riley and his group visited Garscube for just a morning in May 1988. Their report, published in January 1989 produced the devastating news that the Glasgow School was to be merged with the Edinburgh School and a new Scottish School of Veterinary Studies was to be formed and sited mainly in Edinburgh with limited resources made available to house the Glasgow staff and students. The Cambridge School was also threatened with closure.[105]

Save Glasgow Vet School - again!

James Armour, although alarmed, was confident that 'our research record, innovative curriculum and excellent clinical referral service would ensure our future'. The Glasgow spirit kicked in and a massive campaign was mounted to save the School.[106]

Led by Sir William Fraser, the new Principal and James Armour, a huge public awareness campaign was launched which involved the whole of the staff and students at Garscube (and at Gilmorehill) and was supported by the RCVS, politicians across the political divide and the Scottish media. Support was worldwide as the recommendations for closure also prompted a storm of protests from America, Canada, Argentina, Kenya, Morocco, Australia and New Zealand. The response from the people of Glasgow and the West of Scotland was overwhelming. Cars all over Scotland sported 'Evening Times' 'Save the Vet School' stickers.[107]

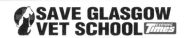

Sir William Fraser, in his response to the Report to the UGC, observed that 'the proposed closure of the Glasgow Veterinary School would have a long term damaging effect on veterinary and allied research in this country.

We believe that the way forward for veterinary education involves the continuation of all six Schools and the creation and development of centres of excellence able to take account of new research developments and techniques to the benefit of the training process, all built around properly funded core teaching augmented by alternative funding'.[108] A petition was launched, supported by the editors of the 'Evening Times' and 'Glasgow Herald', John Scott and Arnold Kemp respectively, and over 700,000 signatures were obtained from the Channel Islands to the Shetlands.

The petition was delivered by James Armour along with Sir William Weipers, who had come out of retirement to lend his support, Sir James Black, Professor Andrew Nash, and Fiona Selkirk, to the Scottish Secretary at Dover House to be presented to the Prime Minister Margaret Thatcher. James Armour was later invited to Downing Street to discuss the Riley Report with the PM herself.

The Government set up another Working Party under Professor Ewan Page to review the manpower requirements of the veterinary profession. The Page Report was published in January 1990, just over a year after the Riley Report. They recommended that the six veterinary schools in the UK should be retained and expanded to meet the increasing demand for vets and both the Glasgow and Cambridge schools survived and flourished.[109,110]

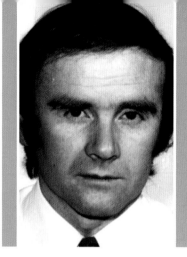

Norman Wright, the seventh Dean, 1991-1999

Norman Wright became Dean in 1991 and continued to move the school forward in the uncertain times post-Riley. Educated at Kilmarnock Academy, he was a Glasgow graduate of 1962, a vintage year as it was the first to avoid the thirty percent failure rate, the accepted result of that era. He then spent a year in practice in Kilmarnock before returning to Buccleuch Street to join the Department of Pathology.

In 1968, he moved to Garscube with Bill Jarrett's hospital pathology group. He carried out seminal work in viral pathogenesis and glomerulonephritis in the dog. He became Professor of Anatomy in 1975 at the age of thirtysix and went on to become the longest serving Dean of recent years, helping to launch the careers of many PhD stars along the way. He held the chair in Veterinary Anatomy until he retired in 2000. Under Norrie's direction, the Vet School flourished.

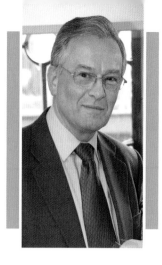

Norman Wright

Andrew Nash

Glasgow moves forward

Under the deanship of Professor Norman Wright the Vet School went from strength to strength.[111] He commented on his time as Dean. 'The most significant event was the creation by the University of a Veterinary Faculty Planning Unit with its own devolved budget. For the first time, this allowed greater autonomy for the Faculty to select its own priorities for development[112] including novel undergraduate and postgraduate training approaches as well as new research initiatives, an imaginative building programme, cutting edge technology transfer, and commercial expansion of diagnostic and clinical services.'

The developments at Garscube were greatly assisted and promoted by the significant, and disproportionate, number of University Vice-Principals from the Vet School. From 1980 onwards a member of the Vet School staff served as a Vice-Principal to each of the five Principals of the University of Glasgow – a record unmatched by any other part of the University. Bill Mulligan (1980-1984) was one of the first Vice-Principals to be appointed to this new post and served Sir Alwyn Williams. This was followed by Sir James Armour's period of Vice-Principal with Sir William Kerr Fraser (1991-96). In 1997 Peter Holmes was promoted to Vice-Principal and served for ten years (1997-2006).

Andrew Nash was elected Clerk of Senate in 2002 and later combined this role with that of Vice-Principal for Learning and Teaching from 2002-2004. He was followed in the role of Vice-Principal for Learning and Teaching by Andrea Nolan in 2004 and in 2009 she became Senior Vice-Principal and Deputy Vice-Chancellor.

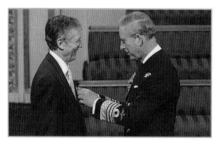

Peter Holmes receiving his OBE 2007

Curriculum contines to evolve

The course was continually evolving, and still is, but one important change to the curriculum took place in the 1991-1992 session, with the formation of a new course, Veterinary Biomolecular Sciences, replacing the previous courses in chemistry and biochemistry. In this session, animal husbandry and management was relabelled veterinary animal husbandry, and therapeutics was brought down into the Third Year. Food hygiene and meat inspection remained within the Fourth Year of the course but were re-branded as veterinary public health.

Clinical Scholars Programme

An innovative Clinical Scholars Programme (CSP) was developed in 1994. The objective was to extend and improve postgraduate training, not only in research but also in the clinical disciplines. Up until the mid-1980s newly qualified vets were given *ad hoc* training as in-service house surgeons or house physicians in veterinary schools. The CSP required new graduates to work not only in service activities but also to participate in formal specialisation training courses to obtain certificates and diplomas, qualifications formally recognised by the RCVS and European Community. Because of the formal training component, the tax authorities accepted the case made by Norman Wright that salaries should be tax-free. As a consequence, many more graduates could be taken on for postgraduate training. In 1985 there were ten house surgeons/physicians; by 2002, this had increased to over thirty clinical scholars and the numbers continue to grow as additional financial resources are identified.

This initiative was taken up by all the other UK veterinary schools and laid the basis of the residency programme that now dominates the profession.

1966
William Weipers receives knighthood.

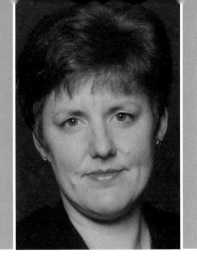

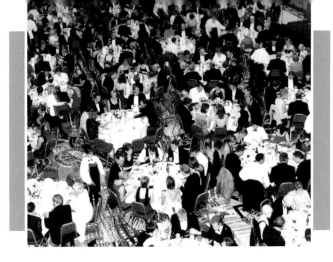

Andrea Nolan　　　　　*Jubilee Banquet at Kelvingrove Art Gallery and Museum*

In 1997 the Departments of Anatomy, Physiology, Histology and Pharmacology merged to form a single Pre-Clinical Division. The clinical departments became the Division of Veterinary Clinical Studies which included Medicine, Surgery, Animal Husbandry and Clinical Biochemistry while Parasitology and Pathology remained separate. The implications of these changes to the pre-clinical and clinical areas of the course were to allow much closer integration of the curriculum and for the clinical teaching to become species orientated.

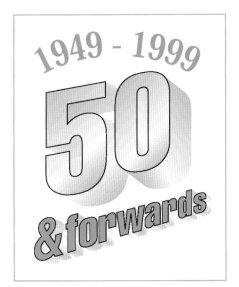

Fifty & Forwards 1949 - 1999 Golden Jubilee celebration

In Dean Andrea Nolan's welcoming speech in 1999 to open the celebrations of the fiftieth anniversary of the amalgamation with the University, she discussed the relationship of the School and the University, 'The position of the Veterinary School under the auspices of a great civic institution that is the University of Glasgow, has allowed the Veterinary School to optimise its potential and develop into the internationally recognised centre of excellence that it is today.

From such a strong all-encompassing base, Glasgow Vet School has been outward in its education and research developments. We have built upon the early collaborations with Institutes and Universities in Africa and we now operate in an international context with links and innovations in every corner of the world'.

The Jubilee Committee organised a celebratory Continuing Professional Development weekend. Celebrations incorporated a busy social and lecture programme. The lecture programme included speakers from home and abroad and covered the wide spectrum of veterinary science.

There were practical demonstrations given by experts in the field which allowed 'hands on' experience while the 'New Horizons programme' gave the brightest young scientists a chance to present their research on 'what's to come'. The social programme had something for everyone: for the delegates and their partners, from sport to shopping, culture and art.

For many, the highlight of the festivities was the banquet held in the magnificent surroundings of the foyer of the Kelvingrove Art Gallery and Museum. Distinguished speakers, Professor Rona Mackie, Dr Bob Michell, Jim Wight and Sir James Armour entertained the audience. A traditional ceilidh rounded off the evening and the dancing continued into the wee small hours. Old friends were reunited and new friendships were forged. The delegates true to form worked hard and played hard![113]

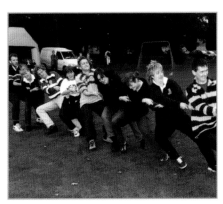

Jubilee celebrations

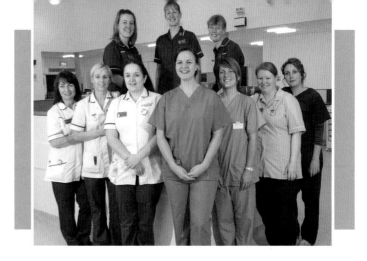

Janis Hamilton, previously a laboratory technician at the Western Infirmary, Glasgow came to the Vet School in 1991. She trained as a nurse at the Vet School and attended night classes there. She comments that there have been many changes in veterinary nursing over the years. The nurse used to have a job first and then undertake training, now the nurse can train and then apply for a job.

The Vet School course (Level 3 Diploma in Veterinary Nursing) is full time and can be converted to a degree in nursing at Napier University. Now nurses can be specialists in physiotherapy, nutrition, surgery and anaesthesia and have greater responsibility.

Veterinary nursing team 2010

Veterinary nursing

The Veterinary School had always been an important training ground for veterinary nurses but as this arm of the veterinary profession developed during the 1990s the training of veterinary nurses became more formalised. Since 1999, in partnership with Telford College in Edinburgh and approved by the RCVS, a full time nursing course has been run by the School. It is a popular course: twentyfour student veterinary nurses are selected from over two hundred applicants and trained over a course of two and a half years. The students attain a consistently higher pass rate than the national average due to the first class facilities and excellent teaching and mentoring by the small animal nursing staff. Many of the students have been employed by the Veterinary School. Formal lectures at Telford College are combined with practical experience in the Small Animal Hospital, on placement and at the Scottish Society for the Prevention of Cruelty to Animals and Riding for the Disabled.[114]

Mike Purton

Joining Veterinary Anatomy in 1977, Mike was a stalwart member of the team and played a leading role in introducing students to the anatomy of exotics and started the School's reptile collection. He retired in 2009. The teaching of 'exotics' and 'small furries' is now very much part of the undergraduate curriculum.

Overseas veterinary students and accreditation

There has been a long tradition of overseas students studying veterinary medicine at Glasgow but details from early years are scant. However, after the First World War, the records are more detailed and indicate that until the merger in 1949, of the 1,151 students who had enrolled, thirtyseven came from overseas.[115] In the 1950s and 1960s there was a steady stream of students from African countries which at that time did not have veterinary schools. Towards the end of the 1960s the newly independent countries of Africa developed their own veterinary schools and the numbers of undergraduates from these countries rapidly diminished. They were replaced, however, by increasing numbers of African postgraduate students. In the new century there have been significant numbers of undergraduates from Botswana, which is one of the few African countries which has preferred to send its students overseas to be trained at the leading veterinary schools.

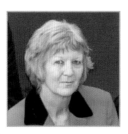

*Joyce Wason
Admissions Manager 2012*

European Association of Establishments for Veterinary Education (EAVE)

During late 1980s a programme of international accreditation of European veterinary schools had been developed by the European Association of Establishments for Veterinary Education (EAVE) and Glasgow was an early School to be accredited in 1989.

In 1991, the 4th General Assembly of EAVE, and the first to be held in the UK, was held at Garscube. Representatives of fifty Veterinary Schools in Europe attended.[116]

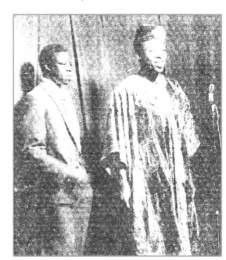

Freshers social, Wally Esuroso and Raymond Oketa 1960s

1966
First ever slow-release intra-ruminal alloy bolus to help prevent magnesium deficiency in cattle is patented by the University of Glasgow.

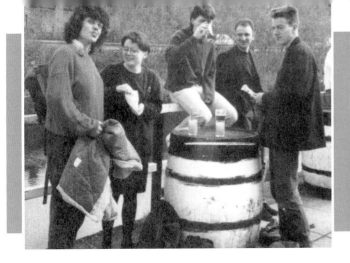

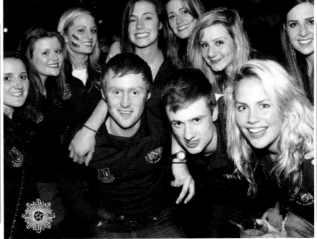

American Veterinary Medical Association (AVMA) Accreditation

To attract student applications from North America it was considered very advantageous for the School to have accreditation from the AVMA. This would mean that our graduates could practice in America without further clinical practice or having to take the Educational Commission for Foreign Veterinary Graduates (ECFVG) examinations. In May 1999, the Veterinary School was visited by officials from the AVMA for inspection and evaluation. At this time only the veterinary schools in London and Utrecht had the prestigious AVMA recognition.

The AVMA representatives spent five days critically evaluating the Vet School on the Garscube Estate. No stones were left unturned; cat kennels to dog wards, cow sheds to equine operating theatres were all inspected; lecturers, residents and students appraised and piles of paperwork perused. The months of preparations, meetings and plans were richly rewarded.

Initial feedback was promising, but after a long wait, the verdict 'approved!' was returned in October of that year. Unqualified approval was awarded for a period of seven years.

The Faculty was congratulated on the high standard of its teaching programme, its quality of staff and students and particularly on the outstanding *esprit de corps*. The approval endorsed the School's excellent teaching, academic record, research and standards of clinical care and recognised Glasgow as a truly 'world class' Vet School.[117]

Following AVMA approval in 1999, the Faculty's association with AVMA was strengthened by their request that the Faculty considered becoming the European Centre for the Clinical Proficiency Examination which is required as part of the ECFVG certification. After a rigorous inspection of the facilities by AVMA, the first diet of examinations was held in June 2002.

In 2007, the Faculty was delighted to announce that it had received re-accreditation from AVMA for another seven years. The Faculty was complimented on its organisational structure and efficient management.

Cochno Farm had undergone renovations and was commended as a valuable resource enabling students to develop animal handling and management and elementary diagnostic skills. Also noted was the opportunity for 'hands on' and 'real life experience' gained through working with the People's Dispensary for Sick Animals, Clyde Veterinary Group and other local practices. Moodle, the University Virtual Learning Environment was highlighted as a unique learning resource.

Further commendations included curricular strengths such as communication skills taught through role play with actors and the recent employment of Objective Structured Clinical Examinations (OSCE) as a form of assessment. Commendations were made to both staff and students.[118]

Student American Veterinary Medical Association

The Student American Veterinary Medical Association (SAVMA) was created in 1969 in the USA and is dedicated to the same objectives as the American Veterinary Medical Association: 'to advance the science and art of veterinary medicine, including its relationship to agriculture and public health.' SAVMA is comprised of twenty nine Chapters at accredited veterinary medical schools in the USA, Canada, and two schools in the Caribbean. With over 10,000 student members, SAVMA 'promotes the exchange of ideas and information, and supports student interests on issues impacting veterinary medicine, not only for North American students, but for the global community at large.' The AVMA requires 60 percent of the student body to become members for the club to become an official chapter. In 2011, Glasgow was able to obtain greater than seventy percent participation, an application for formal recognition was submitted, and in November 2011, the AVMA voted to recognise Glasgow as the first official International Chapter of SAVMA outside the Americas.

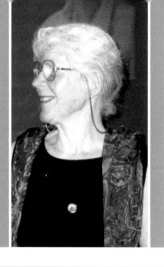

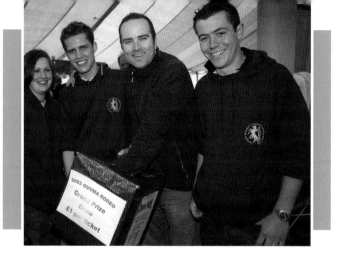

The first 'Rodeo' was given its name by Mary Stewart. She and some friends decided that the school should have an exciting event. Although there was no riding of bucking broncos or steers, they had staff/student competitions including tug-o'-war and donkey races (she remembers Ian McIntyre bobbing along in his kilt). The event continues today on an annual basis. It's a family fun day run by students to raise awareness of animal welfare issues, educate in a fun way and raise money for charity.[119, 120]

Mary Stewart   *Rodeo 2003*

	2002	2003	2004	2005	2006	2007	2008	2009	2010	2011
USA/Canada	18	21	32	33	39	41	32	39	41	43
Botswana	0	0	0	0	2	5	3	9	11	5
Others	3	2	2	0	0	7	5	4	7	14
Total no. overseas students	21	23	34	33	41	53	40	52	59	62

Annual overseas student intake

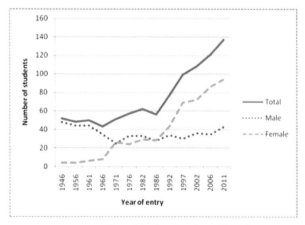

Annual intake of male and female students

Student gender balance

In addition to the marked changes in the ratio of British to non-EU undergraduates the other major change has been the reversal in the gender balance of the undergraduate classes. As the total number of students rose in the 1990s the proportion of female students also rose dramatically so that they now average about seventy percent of the undergraduate students; changed days indeed from the 1930s when the first Scottish female veterinary student graduated from Glasgow.

Modern teaching innovations towards the 21st century

Students from all over the world have chosen to undertake study at the School because of the excellent reputation of its teaching course and the high standing of its graduates. The teaching course is constantly evolving and Glasgow has been at the forefront of innovations in veterinary education from the lecture-free final year to the latest technologies. Glasgow veterinary undergraduates are now taught by methods that could not have been dreamt of by James McCall and his colleagues.

CLIVE and Moodle

E-Learning was introduced when the Computer-aided Learning In Veterinary Education (CLIVE) consortium was established as a Teaching and Learning Technology Programme project in 1993. Glasgow is part of the consortium and has strong links with the other UK veterinary schools.[121] Computer-Assisted Learning has become an established and expanding feature of veterinary undergraduate education in all subjects of the veterinary curriculum.[122]

Gone are the days of blackboards and acetates; instead lectures are uploaded onto 'Moodle' (Modular Object-Oriented Dynamic Learning Environment) a week before they are to take place so that students can go through them in advance. Moodle also includes the facility to upload computer files so that students can submit documents such as essays and reports, via their computer.

Once registered, students can log on from anywhere in the world and retrieve their lecture notes, presentations, videos and other information (including recordings of some lectures!) from all five years of the veterinary programme. McCall may have wondered at what point lectures would still be necessary!

1968
Faculty of Veterinary Medicine established with Sir William Weipers as Dean.

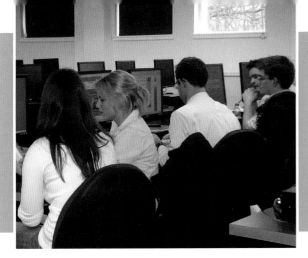
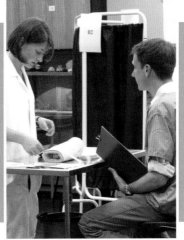
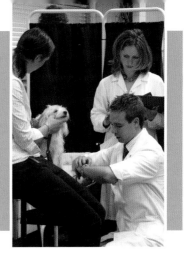

Monitoring of performance of all academic staff is mandatory and students provide constant feedback on staff lectures and tutorials. The students have high expectations and obtaining high scores in the National Student Survey is crucially important to the Veterinary School and the University to continue attracting staff and students from overseas – fortunately these are achieved on an annual basis.[123]

'The Virtual Rectum'

Recent advances have not only changed the lecture delivery but also teaching some of the 'hands-on' clinical skills. One such innovation is known affectionately as 'the virtual rectum'. The Haptic Horse and Haptic Cow, virtual reality simulators, developed to help train veterinary students to palpate an animal's reproductive tract, to perform fertility examinations and to diagnose pregnancy, was first used in teaching in 2003. These were based on the 'virtual rectum' conceived by Professors Brewster, Mellor and Reid in the late 1990s and were developed and validated by PhD students Andrew Crossan and Sarah Baillie.

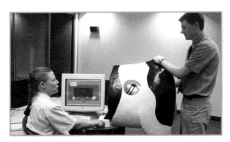

Haptic cow

Finals continue...but with a twist...OSCEs

'Students wait nervously preparing to go into their final exam – sweaty palms and nervous chatter fill the room; this is the culmination of five years of hard graft and intensive learning: who is good enough to become a vet?'

The scene will be a familiar one to anyone who has graduated from the School. The challenge of the final exam is a unique rite of passage into the profession, a chance to demonstrate competency in the basic skills required to begin a career as veterinary surgeon. Indeed the RCVS now specifies a list of 'day-one competencies' required of graduating veterinary surgeons. The challenge for the School is how best to ensure these competencies in its new graduates and the development of the Objective Structured Clinical Examination (OSCE) is a major part of this process.

The OSCE was first developed in Dundee Medical School in the 1970s to assess medical undergraduates and is now used all over the world. The first OSCE to be used in veterinary education was developed by Martin Sullivan and John Mould in 2004 at Glasgow.

An OSCE is an exam composed of a series of short stations between which candidates move. At each station the candidate is asked to demonstrate a specified skill.

The skills assessed are many and varied: for example candidates may be asked to don a surgical gown and gloves in a sterile fashion or to take a history from an owner of an itchy dog, or to make and examine a blood smear.

OSCEs are now integrated throughout the BVMS course and are very much a part of the exams required to be passed to allow progression from year to year.[124]

Mark scheme/model answer	
action/response	**Max**
Introduces him/herself to client	1
Closes the consultation (with reference to phoning if you have questions)	1
General communication skills: establishes rapport, eye contact, non-verbal communication, appropriate language, professional manner, clarity, listening. (to be marked in conjunction with actor)	6
1. Explains that Max has Campylobacter which is a bacterial infection which may be the cause of the diarrhoea	1
2. Explains that this is zoonotic ie can be transmitted to humans	2
Treatment:	
1. Explains that Max will require a full course of antibiotics (erythromycin)	1
2. Explains that erythromycin can sometimes make dogs vomit	1
Identifies that client has 2 children and an elderly mother who come into contact with Max and therefore may be at risk	1
Asks if anyone in the family has diarrhoea	1
Advises client to take affected child to the doctors with a faecal sample	0.5
Identifies that Max is walked off lead in a local park and advises that he should be kept in the garden until the treatment is completed	0.5
In the garden he should be supervised so that all faeces should be collected.	0.5
Children should be kept away from faeces	0.5
Advises client of routine hygiene precautions (wear gloves to pick up poo, hand washing, dealing with soiled materials, do not allow dog to lick humans)	0.5
Advises client not to take Max to visit elderly mother until treatment is completed	1.5
Follow-up: Repeat faecal sample should be collected at end of treatment to confirm Campylobacter has cleared	1
TOTAL	**20**

Candidate ran out of time (please record if this is the case)			
Other comments:			
Fail	**Borderline**	**Pass**	**Good pass**

OSCE mark sheet

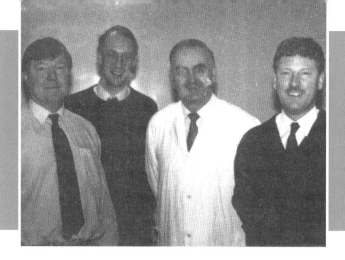

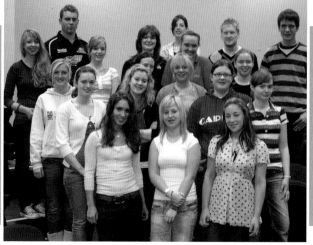

John Anderson, Graham Cochrane, Jack McPhee and Billy Steele 1998

First cohort of Veterinary Biosciences students 2008

New century and new courses

Master of Veterinary Public Health

Glasgow Veterinary School has long been acknowledged as being a centre of excellence in veterinary public health and epidemiology.[125]

The first students were welcomed to a new Master of Veterinary Public Health degree programme in 2006. The programme, originally developed by Dominic Mellor and currently led by Billy Steele, was designed to provide comprehensive training in all aspects of veterinary public health.

Open to veterinary and non-veterinary graduates, it can be studied full- or part-time. The programme provides a rational synthesis of essential subjects of current and growing importance to all those involved at the human–animal interface and in the production and safety of foods of animal origin.[126]

Based on the efforts of Tim Parkin, Lisa Boden, Stuart Reid and Dominic Mellor, the School is one of only four institutions in Europe with a generic training programme in population medicine approved by the European College of Veterinary Public Health.

Official Veterinary Surgeons course

The Faculty was the first organisation in the UK to be approved by the Food Standards Agency (FSA) and Meat Hygiene Service (MHS) to provide Official Veterinarian training. The new course, set up in 2006, was adapted to meet alterations in European Union legislation which changed the way in which veterinary surgeons become designated to work in food premises. It is an intensive three week course which complements the Master's degree programme in veterinary public health and involves food hygiene, pathology, epidemiology and enforcement. It attracts interest from all over Europe and beyond. On completion of the course, vets are eligible for appointment as 'Official Veterinarians' by the MHS and FSA.[127]

Veterinary College Founder, James McCall, with his interests in meat and dairy inspection, would no doubt have approved.

Veterinary Public Health students in all of the School's programmes and courses are also able to access the 'virtual abattoir'. This has been created to meet the need for veterinary students and others to understand the processes which occur in the slaughter of food animals for human consumption and takes the student through each step to maximise understanding and ensure that they are prepared for actual visits or work experience.[128]

Bachelor of Veterinary Biosciences

In 2008, the Faculty established an innovative new degree, the Bachelor in Veterinary Biosciences, with David Barrett as Programme Director. This was the first four-year honours course offered by the Faculty and twenty students were enrolled. The programme is dedicated to the areas of science that underpin veterinary medicine and covers comparative biomedical sciences (anatomy, physiology and biomolecular science), pathological sciences (such as infectious disease and molecular oncology) and the principles and effects of drug action and laboratory diagnostics. The final year includes ethics, animal welfare, population medicine, epidemiology, veterinary public health and a business in bioscience course. Additionally, students undertake a research project chosen from a wide choice of topics. Those students who undertake an industrial placement between years three and four will graduate with the degree of M.Sci.

The programme is designed to provide an outstanding preparation for research studentships, assistantships and fellowships in veterinary research; and for those considering a career in the animal care or pharmaceutical industries.[129, 130] The first cohort of students graduated in July 2012.

1969

The Department of Veterinary Anatomy moves to Garscube and Buccleuch Street closes its doors for the last time.

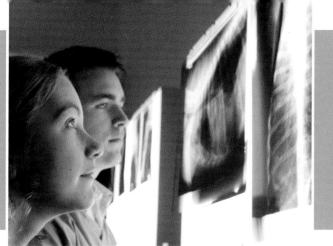
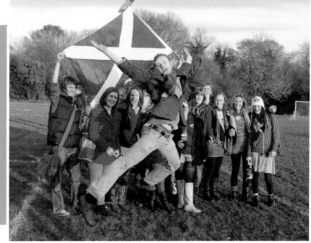

The BVMS programme: into the future

When the College became part of the University of Glasgow in 1949 the professional degree programme of BVMS was born. The BVMS has been the launch pad for thousands of successful careers in all branches of veterinary endeavour and because of the broad training, success in other important arenas. The programme is recognised nationally and internationally both by accrediting bodies and employers for the excellence of its graduates.

To remain at the forefront of the education of veterinary professionals the BVMS programme has changed over the years to respond to the evolving requirements of the profession and society. In 1981 the leaders of the BVMS programme set the bench mark for veterinary education creating the 'lecture-free' final year, signposting the necessity of creating a transition phase for 'soon to be' professionals. Knowledge and developing skills were honed within the supportive educational environment that the University can offer before graduating into the professional environment, ready to take up challenges.

In the last decade the accrediting bodies (RCVS, AVMA and EAEVE) have changed the ethos of accreditation from asking 'what do you teach' to 'this is what we expect of your graduates' as they have moved to competency-based accreditation of professional programmes. During this period the educational environment and technological understanding of staff has changed, as have students and their expectations of their professional education. In a world that is changing, the current custodians of the BVMS programme have to keep veterinary education in Glasgow at the top of the field by responding to the requirements of the accrediting bodies and also asking what skills and knowledge Glasgow graduates need to ensure that they get their career of choice.

Looking to the future, in December 2009 the School of Veterinary Medicine brought together BVMS programme managers, professional bodies, and current students to direct future development of the BVMS programme. The programme was also benchmarked against education in North America and Australia, confirming the ambition of the school to continue to offer an internationally relevant degree. Currently, the School is evolving radical changes to the BVMS programme to provide the optimal educational environment for graduates to meet the needs of the profession and society into the future. The School has looked critically at the teaching in the earlier years of the programme and by rearranging current material and adding new material,

Veterinary Professional and Clinical Skills courses have been created in the first three years to complement the last two clinically orientated years. Students start focusing on their professional development earlier in the programme, meaning greater preparation for Extra Mural Studies and for that essential transition phase to professional status.

Going forward the plan is to broaden the opportunities for students, particularly in Final Year, offering electives that will allow students to develop a level of specialisation such as in pig or poultry medicine. Alternatively, they may choose a short course of particular relevance to them such as the study of tropical diseases.

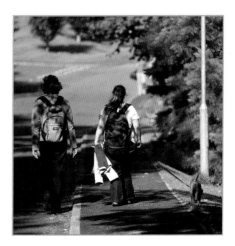

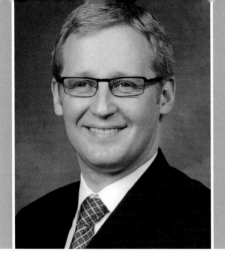

Professor Stuart Reid, Dean of the Faculty (2005-2010) and Head of the new School (2010-2011)

Of particular joy have been the graduations, the innovation of the alumni dinners where we have welcomed back so many friends and former students, and the internationalisation of our Faculty and students. All of these speak louder than any single achievement, representing, as they do the family that is Glasgow Vet School.

For the Faculty is not a building or a title or a programme or a degree, it is the people that make the many good things happen.

It has been a privilege to work with a group of outstanding individuals, whose commitment and energy have developed the organisation we inherited and have made what we now hand on to the next generation and our next chapter. And, reflecting on the accounts... of the other eight deans' terms of office, one realises that, truly, the road to success is always under construction.'

Professor Ewan Cameron, Head of School from 2011

'I was immensely proud to be given this opportunity and to be current custodian of our heritage, but also struck by the deep sense of responsibility that accompanies the position. I will endeavour to maintain the high standards set by my distinguished line of predecessors.'

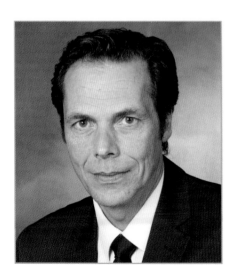

Glasgow Vet School... 150 Years On!

By GUVMA reps for 2012 Rachael Forgie and Susanna Spence What has changed. What hasn't. What is going to change.

A lot has changed in the last 150 years. The campus has moved and grown, facilities have become bigger and better, class sizes have dramatically increased, each year is multinational, the student body is dominated by girls and many great vets and vet students alike have passed through our school. These days the first thing you notice when driving onto Garscube estate is our world class, £15M Small Animal Hospital. In addition, to being able to boast the fact it is one of the best in Europe it also allows our students to experience a high degree of specialism in this modern veterinary world.

However, some things will never change. Glasgow Vets are still the most social students of all the veterinary schools, forming a close knit group that is envied by the rest. Our social calendar reflects this with barely a week going by without a GUVMA event. The old favourites such as AVS, Dick Day, Vet Ball and Rodeo have remained the unmissable events. However, many new traditions have arisen such as 'Mr Vet School' which stirs up much excitement and becomes less and less 'PC' each year. The Hut, once an abandoned shack, is now actually made of bricks. Despite having luxuries such as a kitchen, a plasma screen TV and central heating, don't be fooled!

It is still a student common room and carries with it all the stereotypes you would expect and is still central to our social lives, hosting the infamous 'Hut Parties'. The staff-student relationship is still as strong as ever and although the lecturers may have changed, their characters are still as vibrant and their attendance at parties is still crucial to their success. With these qualities, Glasgow students are extremely well rounded and that is why we are still producing the best vets in the world.

In order to maintain the reputation of being one of the most respected vet schools, Glasgow has to evolve with the times and there are a lot of big changes on the horizon. The curriculum is currently undergoing a massive re-structure, with clinical skills being implemented from day one. Final year is still lecture-free; however, in a couple of years rotations will start in Fourth year and there will be more time spent in first opinion practice. Coinciding with the new curriculum will be a brand new state of the art building, incorporating social areas, study space and support services for our staff and students. The days of paper and pens with printed notes will be a thing of the past with the view to having a paper-free campus. Students will be encouraged to use modern technology such as iPads and Kindles to access lectures and annotate notes. With these changes Glasgow Vet School will undoubtedly continue to thrive and will produce top class vets for years to come. No matter what year students graduate, they will always be proud to be a Glasgow Vet.

1974

Silver Jubilee of the University of Glasgow Veterinary School and the retirement of Sir William Weipers.

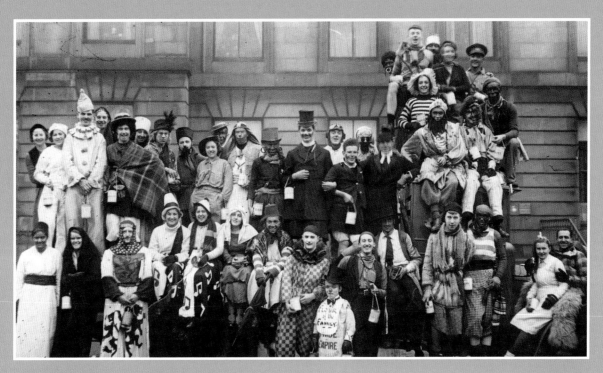

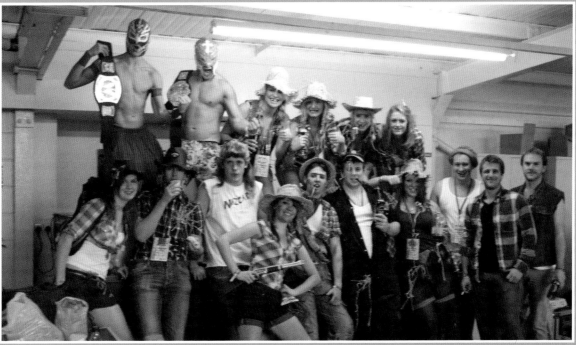

'Some things change... and some things don't'
Top: Charities day 1930s
Bottom: GUVMA party 2012

Chapter Four

Discovery and Innovation

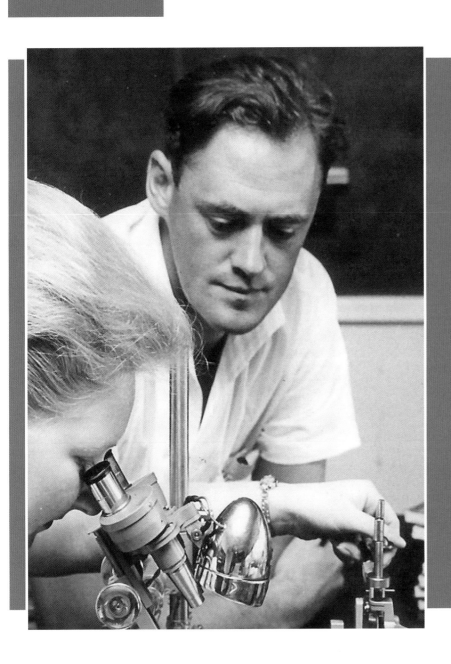

Weipers' vision of 'One Medicine'

With the appointment of William Weipers as Director of the Veterinary School and its amalgamation with the Faculty of Medicine of the University of Glasgow in 1949, research was given a much higher profile. The pathogenesis of many diseases in our animals was largely unknown and methods for treatment and prevention, such as antibiotics and effective vaccines, were sparse and only beginning to appear. At that time few could have anticipated the impact that the School was to have on research and innovation in both animals and man over the following sixty years.

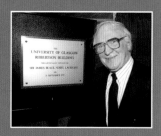
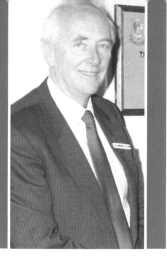
Parasitology

Ruminant helminths

The group that formed to investigate prevalent diseases caused by helminth parasites developed into one of the most formidable and successful parasitology teams in the world over the next sixty years. Their programme involved a unique degree of collaboration among scientists from a wide range of disciplines including clinicians, pathologists, parasitologists, physiologists and biochemists. A powerful study model evolved: an initial detailed description of naturally-occurring outbreaks of disease followed by a sequential analysis of the clinical, pathological and pathophysiological changes produced after experimental infections. Data from these studies provided the template for an understanding of the pathogenesis of the disease and in turn its diagnosis, clinical classification and then the development of a strategy for control or prevention. These principles extended to much of the research in other areas in the School.

Initially three diseases were tackled which were having a massive economic impact on the livestock industry: bovine parasitic bronchitis caused by the lungworm *Dictyocaulus viviparus*; bovine parasitic gastritis caused by the abomasal worm *Ostertagia ostertagi*, and liver fluke in sheep and cattle due to *Fasciola hepatica*. Less comprehensive but original research into infections with *Teladorsagia circumcincta* and *Haemonchus contortus* in sheep was also undertaken, some of the latter work taking place in Kenya.

This research was supported by major funding, first from the main research bodies, most notably by the Agricultural Research Council (later AFRC then BBSRC) and The Wellcome Trust, and through long-term collaboration with international pharmaceutical companies including Allen and Hanburys, Pfizer, Hoechst and Merck, Sharpe and Dohme.

Weipers began by identifying bright young staff, both veterinary surgeons and science graduates, with strong academic records and encouraged them to develop ambitious research programmes. Those recruited included James Black (physiology), George Urquhart (veterinary parasitology), Ian McIntyre (veterinary medicine), Bill Jarrett (veterinary pathology), Bill Mulligan (veterinary physiology) and Frank Jennings (veterinary biochemistry). Weipers' vision of 'One Medicine' which embraced the comparative medicine of man and animals determined the future direction and eminence of the School. Thus, the 1950s saw the new, as well as existing staff at Buccleuch Street (led by Rod Campbell) forming several powerful interdisciplinary research teams.

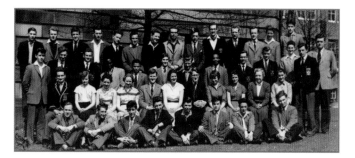

1957-62 year group

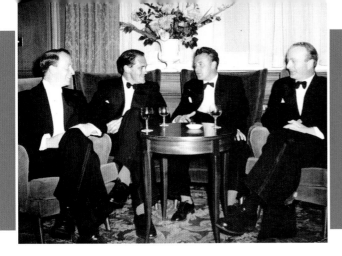
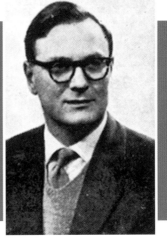
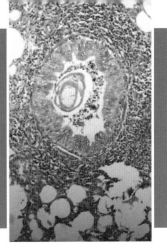

Bill Mulligan, Bill Jarrett, George Urquhart and Ian McIntyre   Frank Jennings   *Dictyocaulus viviparus*, bronchiolitis

Bovine lungworm – the Dictol vaccine

In the early 1950s, George Urquhart turned his attention to parasitic bronchitis which was devastating the cattle population in the UK. He was joined by Ian McIntyre, Bill Mulligan, Frank Jennings, Bill Jarrett, and later pathologist Craig Sharp. Outbreaks were seen mainly in young cattle during their first grazing season and were characterised by severe respiratory problems and frequently death. The disease was commonly referred to as 'Husk' because of the severe coughing.

The group explored the pathogenesis of the causal parasite, the lungworm *Dictyocaulus viviparus*. Following experimental oral infections of calves it was shown that asymptomatic larval migration took place via the intestinal mucosa, mesenteric lymph nodes, blood and lymph, reaching the lungs in about a week.

The pathological changes were incurred during migration in the lungs and increased in severity as the maturing worms reached the main bronchi, inducing severe bronchitis; and in a proportion of calves led to respiratory failure and death. These changes correlated well with the clinical signs seen in the natural field cases.

These experimental studies revealed two significant clues for vaccination: firstly, recovered animals were immune to reinfection, and secondly, the early lung stages caused minimal damage. Hence, it was hypothesised that if infective larvae could be attenuated to a degree that allowed migration to the early lung stages, stimulating an immune response but prior to severe pathology developing, then vaccination against parasitic bronchitis might be feasible.

Bill Mulligan brought to the group considerable expertise in nuclear techniques. Thus a vaccine using ionising radiation to attenuate the larvae of *D. viviparus* was devised. This simple but innovative concept using a unique technique proved to be a major advance in bovine medicine. Following appropriate calibration and the demonstration of a high degree of resistance to challenge, the orally administered vaccine was patented and successfully commercialised in the 1960s as 'Dictol' by Allen and Hanburys.

The first small field trial was carried out on the Bailie Park at Garscube, now the site of The Weipers Centre for Equine Welfare and the new Small Animal Hospital. Ian McIntyre and his secretary Catriona Dunn coordinated the final clinical trials of the vaccine in 8000 calves on 204 farms across Scotland.[134]

Over the past fifty years, millions of cattle have been successfully vaccinated throughout Europe. In 1960, the vaccine was lauded as 'one of the major medical advances of the century' by Sir Harold Himsworth, then secretary of the MRC. Thus, the Dictol group established the Glasgow Veterinary School as a major centre of parasitology research.[135] The lungworm vaccine now marketed as 'Huskvac' was the first, and is still the only successful vaccine against helminth infections in animals or man.[136] The commercial success of Dictol generated substantial royalties that provided long-term support of the School for major research projects, new laboratories, additional staff and postgraduate students.

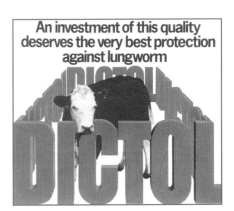

Advert for Dictol

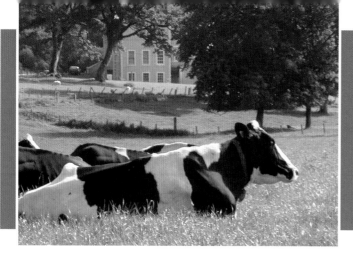

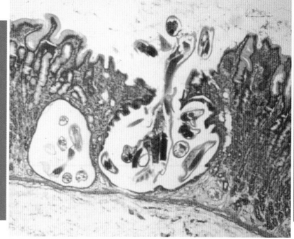

Bovine parasitic gastritis - ostertagiasis

In the 1960s the parasitology team led by George Urquhart was joined by James Armour who, along with Max Murray (pathology), Jim Dargie and Peter Holmes (physiology), Norman Anderson (medicine), Ken Bairden and Ian Maclean (research technologists), conducted seminal work over the next two decades on the other two of the three parasitic diseases which were decimating the cattle and sheep industry in Europe.

Ostertagia ostertagi, like lungworm, has a direct life cycle involving a free-living phase, larval development to the infective third stage and a parasitic maturing phase in the abomasum. Investigation of naturally-occurring outbreaks of ostertagiasis identified two clinical forms primarily seen in dairy herds. The more common Type I disease was usually found in calves grazed intensively during their first grazing season, and occurred from mid-summer onwards. Using these data and through collaboration with George Gettinby at Strathclyde University, a mathematical model was developed which accurately predicted the timing of outbreaks.

A less common but very important second form in housed cattle, Type II, was identified for the first time. This form was seen in yearlings, occasionally in heifers, in late winter or early spring following their first grazing season.

It had previously been recognised as 'winter diarrhoea syndrome' of unknown origin. In fact, it resulted from the maturation of a massive accumulation of fourth stage larvae seasonally arrested (hypobiosis/inhibition) during the previous autumn in the gastric glands. At necropsy, the picture was of a unique hyperplastic nodular gastritis which, particularly in Type II, had a dramatic Morocco leather-like appearance.

Contemporaneous and original experimental studies with oral infections of *O. ostertagi* larvae explained the reasons for the above clinical signs. Following infection the larvae pass to the abomasum where they develop in the gastric glands before moulting twice and emerge to lie on the surface of the gastric mucosa and mature as adults. The worms cause a functional reduction in the gland mass responsible for the production of acidic gastric juice, with pH rising from three to seven. This leads to failure to activate pepsinogen to pepsin and a loss of bacteriostatic effect with a logarithmic increase in bacterial population. At the same time, enhanced permeability of the gastric epithelium to macromolecules is evidenced by hypoalbuminaemia.

The novel finding of elevated plasma pepsinogen levels resulted in the development of a highly specific blood test by Frank Jennings and colleagues, which revolutionised the diagnosis of Type II ostertagiasis when the traditional faecal egg count methods were unreliable.

Many of the foregoing studies led by George Urquhart and Jimmy Armour were carried out in collaboration with several large pharmaceutical companies. New powerful broad spectrum anthelmintics were being developed and strong collaborations were developed with Pfizer (Peter McWilliam – Paratect bolus), Hoescht (David McBeath – benzimidazoles) and Merck, Sharpe and Dohme (John Davidson and Ian Sutherland – benzimidazoles, and John Preston and Dennis Hagen – ivermectin). The detailed knowledge from the Glasgow research of the epidemiology and precise understanding of the disease and its diagnosis, allowed optimal use of these drugs not only for effective treatment but also enabled highly successful strategic prophylactic programmes to be introduced and sustained. However, drug resistance is now a growing problem and new regimes have been developed by scientists at the Moredun Research Institute and elsewhere to slow down resistance and limits its occurrence.

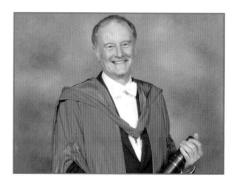

John Preston receiving Honorary degree 2007

1975
Chair of Veterinary Anatomy established.

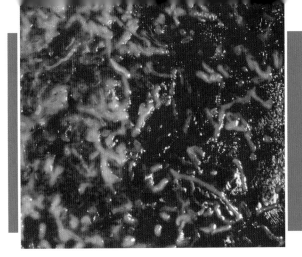

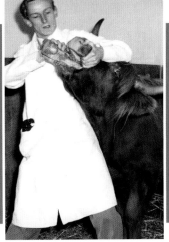

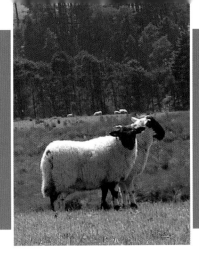

Fasciola hepatica larval tracts in liver   *Dosing sick Highland cow*   *Blackface sheep*

Liver fluke disease in sheep and cattle

In the 1970s, the Glasgow team, now joined by Jimmy Reid, and later George Mitchell turned their attention to the liver fluke *Fasciola hepatica* which was devastating sheep flocks and having a widespread impact on the cattle industry in parts of the UK.

Liver fluke, unlike the bovine lungworm and stomach worms, has an indirect lifecycle involving the mud snail *Lymnaea truncatula* and consequently a more complex epidemiology.

In field studies, acute, sub-acute and chronic forms of fascioliasis were clearly identified. The acute form presented as sudden deaths during autumn and early winter. The sub-acute form, seen mainly in early to mid-winter, presented as a severe anaemia with hypoalbuminaemia leading to a high mortality two to three weeks later. In surviving cases, the enlarged livers were palpable and ascites was present. The chronic form was the most common and occurred in late winter or early spring. Clinical signs included weight loss, pale mucous membranes due to anaemia and hypoalbuminaemia sometimes reflected in submandibular oedema.

These clinical classifications were confirmed from fluke burdens in tracer lambs grazing on pastures previously associated with outbreaks of fascioliasis. All three clinical forms identified in the field were successfully reproduced by dose response studies in experimental infections.

In cattle, extensive field studies showed that the chronic disease was the most common form. Acute or sub-acute disease was rare and confined to very young stock. The time of onset and the pathogenesis was similar to that in sheep but a notable difference was the dramatic calcification of the dilated bile ducts and enlarged gall bladders. Anaemia and hypoalbuminaemia, again defined by radioactive isotope kinetics, were consistent features. A loss of body condition varied according to the level of nutrition.

In some outbreaks, chronic fascioliasis was complicated by the concurrent presence of *Ostertagia* infections with diarrhoea being a feature. In pure infections with liver fluke, the latter was usually not the case. This previously unidentified syndrome was termed the fascioliasis/ostertagiasis Complex.

Based on these studies, highly effective control strategies were devised based on the elimination of snail habitats by improving field drainage, and/or by prophylactic medication linked to predictions of weather patterns suitable for snail development. In this way the reliability of the timing for prophylaxis was greatly improved.

Other important gastric nematodes of sheep

From the 1950s onwards the Glasgow team also carried out pioneering research on the abomasal nematodes *Teladorsagia (Osteragia) circumcincta* and *Haemonchus contortus*.

Studies on *T. circumcincta* found a similar seasonal pattern to that which occurred with *Ostertagia ostertagi* in cattle although the severity of the clinical disease was less dramatic. The same pathological and biochemical changes were evident. The blood-sucking abomasal parasite *H. contortus* is generally considered to be the most important abomasal parasite in ruminants in sub-tropical and tropical areas. Field studies in sheep undertaken by George Urquhart and Ed Allonby in Kenya identified two forms of clinical haemonchosis. The first was an acute syndrome characterised by severe anaemia, with various degrees of oedema and often dark blood-stained faeces. Heavy experimental infections produced similar clinical signs with a severe haemorrhagic gastritis and high mortality two to three weeks after infection. Sometimes in very heavy infections sudden death ensued. The chronic, more common form was most prevalent during the dry season. Control of both ovine ostertagiasis and haemonchiasis was, and still is, dependent on the prophylactic use of anthelmintics integrated where possible with pasture rotation. This worked well although less so in recent years due to widespread development of resistance to the available anthelmintics.

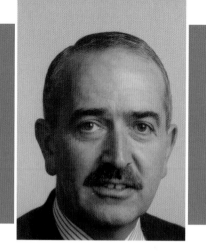
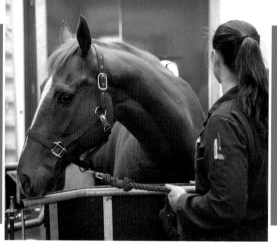
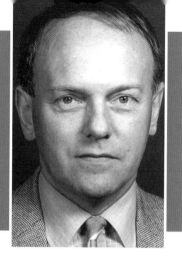

Jimmy Duncan   Weipers Centre for Equine Welfare   Hugh Pirie

Equine helminths

During the 1970s and 1980s similar studies were carried out in equines to those previously conducted in ruminants. These investigations led to the definition of the lifecycles and the characterisation of the pathogenesis of three of the four major equine intestinal parasites in the developed world. Before the advent of modern anthelmintics, *Strongylus vulgaris* was a prevalent and highly pathogenic parasitic infection associated with severe and often fatal colic. Original studies on the definition of the life cycle of this parasite by Jimmy Duncan and Hugh Pirie were key to developing methods for its control: it has a long, migratory parasitic phase during which it is highly susceptible to the action of modern anthelmintics such that it is easy to control to the point where it now rarely occurs in countries in which such drugs are available.

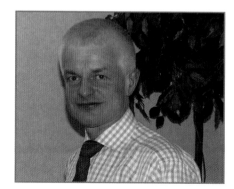

Sandy Love

Subsequently, similar studies were conducted on *Parascaris equorum* by Hilary Clayton and on the cyathostomes (small strongyles). The latter group is now considered to be the principal parasite of equidae and was investigated by Sandy Love.

Two aspects of their biology were shown to be crucial to their pathogenicity and control. First, they have the propensity for undergoing protracted (several years) arrested development within the large intestinal mucosa, then during emergence cause severe protein losing enteropathy.

During the phase of arrested development the cyathostomes have a very low susceptibility to modern anthelmintics and hence are extremely difficult to control. Secondly, they readily develop resistance to the action of all classes of modern broad spectrum anthelmintics. A collaborative study involving the School and the Moredun Research Institute is ongoing to tackle the molecular basis of cyathostome drug resistance.

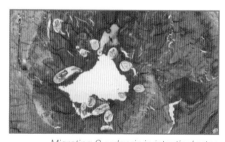

Migrating S. vulgaris in intestinal artery

Basic mechanisms of immunity to intestinal parasites

A key part of the nematode research programme was to explore the fundamental mechanisms by which the host becomes resistant to infection. For this new approach, George Urquhart, Bill Jarrett and Bill Mulligan turned to a laboratory model: the intestinal nematode, *Nippostrongylus brasiliensis*, in its natural host, the rat.

In 1965, they discovered that adult worms were expelled immunologically (self cure) in a predictably exponential fashion and there was an associated intestinal permeability (leak lesion). Ellen Barth (later Ellen Jarrett), George Urquhart and colleagues then extended these findings. In a seminal study they showed that the leak lesion, caused by intestinal anaphylaxis, permitted the passage of anti-worm antibodies into the gut lumen which promoted worm elimination. Between 1966 and 1971, Ellen and George demonstrated very clearly the unresponsiveness of baby rats and its well established similarity and thus relevance, to the equally poor responses in young ruminants.

1977
Bill Mulligan succeeds Ian McIntyre as Dean.

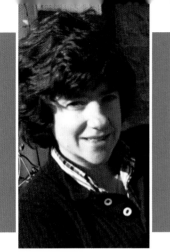

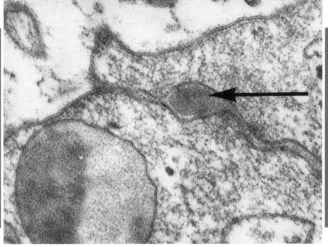

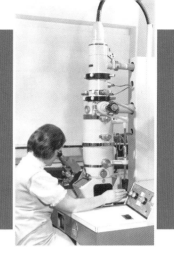

Ellen Jarrett | *Electron microscopy showing 'leak lesion'* | *Electron microscope*

In the following ten years with funding from the Royal Society, The Wellcome Trust and the MRC, Ellen and her colleagues made a detailed analysis of the induction and regulation of the IgE that is massively potentiated by helminth infection. Her work in this field was internationally recognised as pioneering, especially with regard to the maternal regulation of IgE: they suggested that suppression of IgE antibody by maternal IgG has evolved to inhibit the development of infantile allergies.

In complementary studies in rats and ruminants, Hugh Miller, Max Murray and Bill Jarrett explored the mechanisms in the gut that caused the leak lesion. They showed that there was a very substantial recruitment of subepithelial mast cells into the mucosa with the release of mast cell-derived amines, which were involved in the elimination of parasites. Overall, the work resulted in the first cohesive concept of the role of the allergic response in the immune rejection of gut nematodes.

In the early 1980s, Ellen, in her new laboratory built with funds from the MRC and working with David Haig, Christine McMenamin and Lizzie Gault, adopted new *in vitro* approaches to analysing allergy. Ellen's burgeoning and enduring contribution to our understanding of allergic diseases in general, and to helminth immunity, particularly in regard to the development of potential vaccines against small intestinal parasites of domestic animals, was tragically cut short by her untimely death in 1985.

Pathophysiology of parasitic infections

Bill Mulligan's expertise in the use of nuclear techniques, which were applied in the development of the irradiated bovine lungworm vaccine 'Dictol', resulted in recognition of the Vet School as a centre of excellence in the use of nuclear techniques especially for the study of the pathophysiology and control of parasites. This expertise was shared with others through regular courses which Bill Mulligan, Frank Jennings and Ian MacLean ran at Buccleuch Street, and later at Garscube, on nuclear techniques and the use of radioisotopes. With the recruitment of Peter Holmes and Jim Dargie to the Department of Veterinary Physiology in 1966 these nuclear tracer techniques were developed and applied, for the first time, over the next two decades to investigate the underlying pathogenesis of a wide range of parasitic diseases in domestic animals, to quantify changes in protein, red cell and host metabolism. Key outputs were the quantification of the protein losses in the gastrointestinal tract (the so called 'protein-losing gastroenteropathies') and quantification of the dynamic changes in the erythrokinetics and red cell distribution associated with parasitic anaemias.

Peter and Jim, together with Jim Parkins, Jimmy Armour and others, highlighted the central role of changes in protein metabolism and the key impact of nutrition in parasitic infections.

Following Dictol's success a major research programme was initiated to determine whether irradiation could be used to develop other vaccines for parasitic diseases in animals and possibly in man. Varying degrees of immunity were induced by the use of irradiated larvae and in some cases successful vaccines were produced. Tom Miller developed an irradiated vaccine for hookworm disease in dogs caused by *Ancylostoma caninum*, which was marketed the in USA but was subsequently withdrawn for economic reasons. Other notable successes were achieved with *Dioctycaulus filaria* in sheep and *Syngamus trachea* in chickens by visiting scientists in Glasgow, Milovan Jovanovic and Istvan Varga. However, practical problems restricted application in the field. These included the requirement for large numbers of live larvae to be produced in donor animals, the need to vaccinate animals before they had been exposed to natural infections, and the necessity for continuous refrigeration to maintain the living vaccines under field conditions, a problem particularly relevant in developing countries. Nevertheless, attenuation by X-irradiation remains the gold-standard for evaluating new attempts to develop vaccines against a range of parasitic diseases.

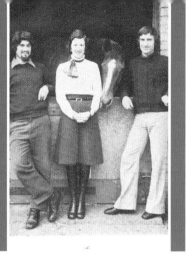

Jim Bogan was tragically killed in an accident in 1988. In 1990 a donation from his family founded the Jim Bogan prize which is awarded annually to a student at the Veterinary School who has excelled in both academic work and sport.

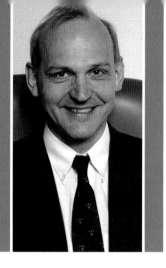

Quintin McKellar BVMS 1981

Quintin McKellar took up the post of Vice-Chancellor of the University of Hertfordshire in 2011. Prior to that he was Principal of the Royal Veterinary College for a period of six years having been the Director of the Moredun Research Institute and Professor of Veterinary Pharmacology at the University of Glasgow. Professor McKellar is also an accomplished rower who represented Scotland in the 1986 Commonwealth games.

David Snow, Grace McKenzie and Jim Bogan 1970s

Quintin McKellar

Pharmacokinetics of anti-parasite drugs

Through pioneering work by Jim Bogan and later by Quintin McKellar the School became a centre of excellence in the pharmacokinetics of anti-parasite drugs.

In 1980, Jim Bogan and Sue Marriner developed a method for the analysis of benzimidazole anthelmintics by high performance liquid chromatography which they used to determine the basic pharmacokinetic characteristics of these drugs in livestock and in man. Further detailed work on the role of the rumen in the absorption and metabolism of what were the 'modern' benzimidazoles resulted in a fuller understanding of the improved efficiency of these anthelmintics compared to their predecessors.

Substantial interspecies differences were noted, and dosing regimens were optimised according to pharmacokinetic characteristics. Similar studies were carried out with ivermectin upon its introduction in 1980 and the high lipophilicity of this drug and its persistence at therapeutic levels in animals allowed the development of integrated dosing strategies which provided whole-season protection of farm livestock.

Quintin McKellar joined the group in 1984 and in subsequent work began to integrate the pharmacokinetics of anthelmintics with their pharmacodynamics. Inhibitors were utilised to reduce the metabolic breakdown of benzimidazoles thereby improving their efficiency and enhancing their effectiveness against nematodes which had developed resistance. These integrated kinetic-dynamic studies pioneered in anthelmintics were extended to antibiotics and anti-inflammatory drugs. During the twenty year period from 1977 strategies for the optimisation of dosage for individual species according to specific pharmacokinetics were implemented and studies with antibiotics were undertaken to characterise the relationships between bacterium, drug and host. This work led to major improvements in the use of these drugs in the livestock industry with greater efficiency and sustainable use, and minimised the risk of resistance in target and commensal organisms.

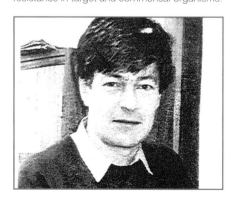

Andy Tait

Molecular biology of parasites

By the late 1980s, despite the successful development of Dictol and the availability of new effective anthelmintic drugs, hopes for further vaccines were not realised and drug resistance had progressively increased. New approaches were required; these are becoming available as a result of developments in genetics and molecular biology.

In 1987, The Wellcome Trust, which was urging more vets to be trained in molecular biology, awarded a grant of £1M to Andy Tait and Dave Barry to establish the Wellcome Unit of Molecular Parasitology (WUMP), the first such unit in the UK. It was located jointly in Veterinary Parasitology at Garscube and the Department of Genetics at Gilmorehill, to link veterinary and biological sciences. The mission of WUMP was to identify and characterise the genes and their associated pathways that govern essential processes in parasites with a view to exploiting that knowledge to develop new methods of disease control. Major funding for the Unit (subsequently designated The Wellcome Trust Centre for Molecular Parasitology) from a wide variety of sources has continued to this day. The influx of funding and high quality scientists enhanced and extended research on parasites in the University as a whole and led to the University of Glasgow being one of the largest parasitology groupings in the world.

1980

Unique multiple trace element/vitamin intra-ruminal device (All-Trace) is patented (Hemingway, Parkins & Ritchie) and now in use worldwide

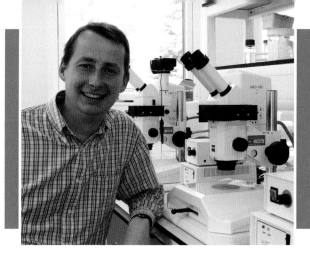
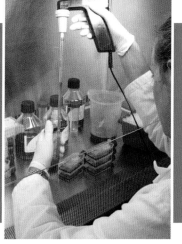
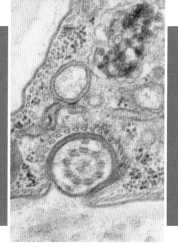

John Gilleard   Cell culture   EM trypanosome brucei brucei

The starting point for understanding the genetic basis of any organism is to obtain the nucleotide sequence of the whole genome. Collaborating with The Wellcome Trust Sanger Institute in Cambridge, the Glasgow parasitologists played key roles in deriving the complete sequences of three species of trypanosome (Andy Tait and Dave Barry), several species of Leishmania (Jeremy Mottram) and the major tropical cattle parasite, *Theileria annulata* (Brian Shiels and Andy Tait). *Haemonchus contortus* (John Gilleard), Plasmodium (Andy Waters) and Toxoplasma (Marcus Messner) are currently being sequenced. In terms of endemic UK disease, research has concentrated on *Haemonchus contortus* and *Teladorsagia circumcincta* with strong collaborative links with the Moredun Research Institute.

Research on tropical parasites, in keeping with the Veterinary School's links with Africa, is focussed on the main protozoan parasites affecting domestic livestock and humans. Trypanosomes are one group that seriously restrain livestock rearing and development, particularly in sub-Saharan Africa. A key feature of trypanosomes is their ability to switch their surface glycoprotein coat from one type to another and so evade the host immune response. Based on their genome sequence and a series of experimental analyses, a mechanism for this antigenic switching was discovered (Dave Barry).

A further highlight has been the analysis of the diversity between different strains of trypanosomes, in particular the zoonotic species group *Trypanosoma brucei*. Using a combination of highly variable molecular markers (identified from the genome sequence) and crosses between parasite strains, Andy Tait, Mike Turner and Annette MacLeod have discovered that the parasite has a sexual cycle which can be exploited to map the genes that determine traits of importance for the transmission, severity and treatment of the disease. Another tropical protozoan parasite which causes high levels of morbidity and mortality is *Theileria parva*. Brian Shiels and Andy Tait have made considerable progress towards developing a sub-unit vaccine by identifying two Theileria antigens that confer significant levels of protection in cattle.

Research on nematodes of veterinary significance has ranged from detailed studies of specific genes and their function, through genomics into genetics and molecular epidemiology. A key feature of the work has been the pioneering use of the closely related free living nematode *Caenorhabditis elegans*. Eileen Devaney, Collette Britton and Tony Page have tested the function and regulation of specific parasite genes, as well as using this system to express Haemonchus antigens as a route to produce a sub-unit vaccine.

In addition, using a combination of genetic and molecular approaches the biochemical pathways that lead to the assembly of collagen, a unique component of the cuticle of these worms, have been identified and characterised; potentially these can be exploited as drug targets.

In a study of drug resistance in Haemonchus, John Gilleard developed genetic markers for detecting drug resistant worms. In addition, analysis of data collected in a UK-wide survey of ovine nematodes has demonstrated that, for at least one class of anthelmintic, resistance arises only a few times and is then spread by livestock movement. These findings are highly significant for planning strategies to contain and reduce the impact of drug resistance.

Thus, Glasgow remains at the forefront of parasitology research internationally through these new developments in molecular biology which are leading to novel methods of diagnosis, treatment and control.

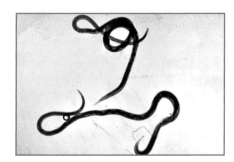

Haemonchus contortus

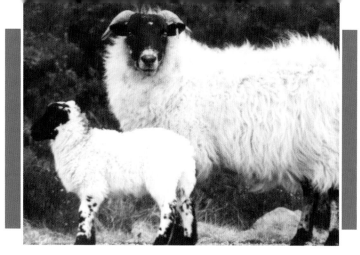

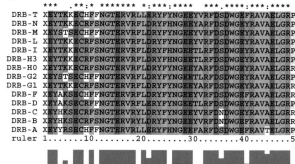

```
            ***  .**:* ******* *:***:****  ***.****:***:****
DRB-T   XEYTKKECHFFNGTERVRLLERYFYNGEEYVRFDSDWGEFRAVAELGRP
DRB-N   XRYTKKECRFSNGTERVRFLDRYFHNGEEYARFDSDWGEYRAVAELGRP
DRB-M   XEYSTSECHFFNGTERVRFLDRYFYNGEEYVRFDSDWGEYRAVAELGRP
DRB-L   XEYTKKECRFSNGTERVRFLDRYFYNGEEYVRFDSDWGEYRAVAELGRP
DRB-I   XEYTKKECRFSNGTERVRFLDRYFHNGEETLRFDSDWGEYRAVAELGRP
DRB-H3  XEYTKKECRFSNGTERVRFLDRYFHNGEETLRFDSDWGEYRAVAELGRP
DRB-H0  XEYTKKECRFSNGTERVRFLDRYFYNGEEYARFDSDWGEYRAVAELGRP
DRB-G2  XEYSTSECHFFNGTERVRFLDRYFYNGEETLRFDSDWGEYRAVAELGRP
DRB-G1  XEYTKKECRFSNGTERVRFLDRYFYNGEEYARFDSDWGEYRAVAELGRP
DRB-F   XEYAKSECHFFNGTERVRFLDRYFYNGEEYVRFDSDWGEFRAVAELGRR
DRB-D   XEYAKSECRFFNGTERVRFLERYFYNGEETLRFDSDWGEYRAVAELGRP
DRB-C   XEYHKSECRFSNGTERVRFLDRYFYNGEEYVRFDNDWGEYRAVAELGRR
DRB-B   XEYHKSECRFSNGTERVRYLDRYFYNGEEYVRFDNDWGEFRAVAELGRR
DRB-A   XEYYRSECHFFNGTERVRLLERYFHNGEEFARFDSDWGEFRAVTELGRR
ruler   1.......10........20........30........40.......5
```

Genetic resistance to helminth infections

The School's interest in genetic resistance of sheep to gastric helminths began when Max Murray in 1985 initiated a long-term project with George Urquhart to follow up the work of John Preston and Ed Allonby (both Glasgow graduates) who had demonstrated significant resistance to *Haemonchus contortus* in indigenous Red Maasai sheep in Kenya in the late 1970s. Also, research on trypanotolerance indicated the likelihood of differences in susceptibility to helminthiasis in various ruminants across Africa.

Mike Stear, joined the group in Glasgow to work on genetic resistance to helminths. He and many colleagues collaborated in Kenya and in Glasgow with major funding from DFID, the EC, BBSRC and The Wellcome Trust. Work was carried out initially in Kenya on *H. contortus* and then in Glasgow on *T. circumcincta*, in local breeds of sheep, mainly Scottish Blackface and Texel. Field and experimental studies demonstrated remarkable within-breed variation in faecal egg output. Using this marker, resistance was found to be heritable. At the same time, it was shown to be favourably genetically correlated with growth rate; resistant animals grew faster.

The basic mechanisms of resistance appeared to be related to two components of the immune response: a local IgA response associated with decreased parasite growth and reduced fecundity, and a local immediate hypersensitivity reaction related to the expulsion of worms from the gastrointestinal tract.

As gastrointestinal worms cannot be counted or measured directly, complementary research looked for additional ways to identify resistant sheep.

Existing biomarkers were quantified and new markers were discovered. Markers include molecules such as pepsinogen, fructosamine, IgA and IgE as well as genes such as DRB1 within the major histocompatibility complex on chromosome 20 and the interferon-gamma gene on chromosome 3. Both genes have strong and consistent effects on resistance to nematode infection. The function of DRB1 molecules gene is to recognise parasites and activate the immune response while the interferon-gamma molecules determine the type of immune response. Results suggest that sheep can be bred for resistance to nematodes and that resistant sheep will have improved productivity.

Once again, the Glasgow interdisciplinary study model has proved its worth as it has moved towards genetics, offering an additional approach for the control of major parasitic diseases of domestic animals.

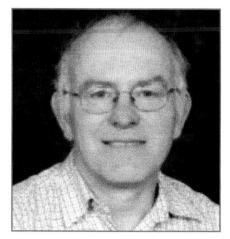

Mike Stear

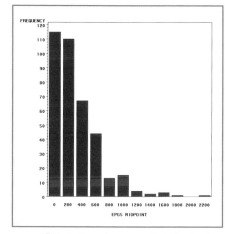

Distribution of egg counts in September in a flock of Blackface

1981
The introduction of a lecture-free final year at Glasgow.

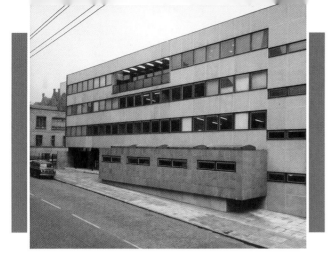

Institute of Virology building, Church Street 1961

Virology

Investigation of infectious diseases was a focus in the Veterinary College from Gaiger's time but it was not until the incorporation of the College into the University, with the recruitment of more specialised staff, that significant advances were made in defining the clinical features, pathology and causes of prevalent viral diseases. The success of these studies was due in large part to the collaborative approach that became the hallmark of research in the School. In this way the causes of several important viral diseases of farm and domestic animals were discovered. As well as controlling these diseases, concepts from this work had remarkable consequences for comparative medicine and led to the establishment of important new areas of study, as in molecular oncology, and the recent siting of one of the largest virology research units in the UK on the Garscube campus.

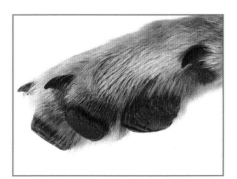

Hardpad due to canine distemper virus

Early research in virology

The study of virology at the new Veterinary School began with research to understand the causes and pathogenesis of diseases that were common in domestic animals at the time. In the urban environment of Glasgow in the 1950s canine distemper was a serious problem in dogs attending the Dog and Cat Free Clinic in the city centre, which was staffed by clinicians from the School, led by Ian Lauder. A detailed clinico-pathological study of cases of distemper by Ian, Bill Martin (then a clinician), Rod Campbell and colleagues in 1954 defined the condition in detail and drew attention to the similarities of distemper, measles and rinderpest. They also determined that the clinical condition of 'hardpad' was part of the distemper syndrome and not a separate condition likely to be caused by another agent, as had been suggested by others.

In the same period, working at the new Veterinary Hospital at Garscube, the pathologists Charles Dow and Bill Jarrett together with Ian McIntyre, described for the first time a disease of cattle in Britain resembling the bovine virus diarrhoea-mucosal disease complex previously reported in the USA, and drew particular attention to the occurrence of abortions in some infected pregnant cows. Attempts to transmit the infection to calves were successful, producing fever and diarrhoea but not fatal mucosal disease.

Although this work was not taken further in Glasgow, it was an indication that the virus, now known as bovine viral diarrhoea virus, produced different conditions in cattle. Virology research then continued on both sites. At Garscube, feline virology became established in a temporary laboratory after the discovery of feline leukaemia virus in 1964. In 1969 the long-delayed new building to house pre- and paraclinical departments from Buccleuch Street was completed and for the first time the virologists working on canine and feline viruses were housed together, with great benefits for both although they continued to collaborate with pathologists and clinicians through two distinct research networks, the Canine Infectious Diseases Unit (CIDRU) and the Feline Virus Unit. Both developed a commercial wing, offering diagnostic support and advice to large numbers of veterinary practitioners throughout the UK and continental Europe, and to industry.

These endeavours provided an immensely valuable contact with conditions in the field as well as a source of funding to support research and development of new diagnostic tests. Eventually the two units merged to form Companion Animal Diagnostics, which also incorporated elements of clinical pathology, and finally became incorporated into Veterinary Diagnostic Services.

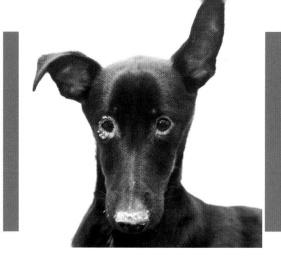

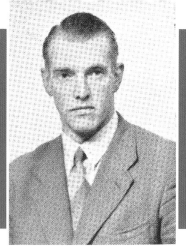

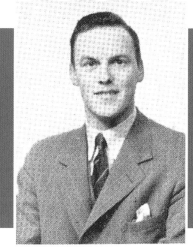

Canine distemper | Ian Lauder | Bill Martin

Canine virology

Canine distemper virus

The timing of the original canine distemper study was fortunate as it coincided with the advent of modern virology and the development of routine cell culture which allowed viruses to be grown and analysed in the laboratory. John Vantsis, a member of staff, was dispatched to the laboratory of Alan Betts in Cambridge to learn the methods and then introduced this new technique to the study of canine distemper virus (CDV) in the School at Buccleuch Street. In 1959 he reported the isolation of CDV from local cases of distemper in cell cultures derived from dogs and ferrets, the first time the virus had been grown in mammalian cells. The group also discovered that CDV caused serious, destructive and suppressive effects on the immune system that allowed the activation of the latent protozoan parasite *Toxoplasma gondii*. Bill Hutchison, a zoology graduate of the University of Glasgow, who studied the parasite in cats at the University of Strathclyde, showed for the first time that it had a natural life cycle based in the cat. He demonstrated that the domestic cat was an important vector of the disease by passing the parasite in its faeces. His findings led to a series of recommended public health measures aimed at creating greater public awareness of the problem.

After John Vantsis left for a senior position at the Moredun Research Institute, research on CDV was continued by Campbell Cornwell and extended to include other emerging viral infections of dogs, in collaboration with the pathologists John Hamilton, Norman Wright, Hal Thompson, Irene McCandlish and Lawson Macartney. CIDRU became a major international centre of dog virology, making pioneering contributions to research on CDV, canine herpesvirus (CHV), canine adenovirus (CAV), canine parainfluenza virus (CPIV) and canine parvovirus (CPV).

Other canine respiratory diseases

The initial mission of the group was to isolate viruses from dogs suffering from conditions that might be of viral origin and then determine their aetiological significance in pathogenesis experiments. Methods were explored to establish optimal conditions for growing the viruses in cell culture and to develop serological tests for diagnosis.

In 1966 Campbell Cornwell, simultaneously with Jack Prydie, another Glasgow veterinary graduate working at the Burroughs Wellcome company, isolated a novel canine herpesvirus (CHV) from cases of a fading puppy syndrome characterised by focal necrosis in many organs.

Further extensive studies in collaboration with Norman Wright defined the pathogenesis of the condition and found that very young pups

were particularly susceptible because the virus replicates at their lower deep body temperature compared to adults. Later they showed that the virus could cause respiratory disease in older pups or adult dogs but it was not likely to be an important cause of respiratory problems, which was a major focus of the group.

At this time John Hamilton published a definitive, detailed study of the pathogenesis of canine viral hepatitis (Rubarth's disease) caused by CAV-1. Further work by Norman Wright showed that two immune-mediated nephropathies, glomerulonephritis and focal interstitial nephritis, persisted in dogs for more than forty days after CAV-1 infection. These results supported, but did not prove, suggestions by others that the virus might also be associated with chronic interstitial nephritis, a common condition in dogs. This work was then extended into developing experimental models for immune complex glomerulonephritis that resembled naturally-occurring membranous nephropathy, the most common immune complex mediated glomerulonephritis in dogs; and with Andrew Nash, immune complex glomerulonephritis and nephrotic syndrome in cats.

The original studies of infectious hepatitis caused by CAV-1 were followed over the next seven years by a series of studies by the group to investigate whether this virus could also cause respiratory disease. The conclusion was that CAV-1 could indeed cause bronchopneumonia following experimental or natural infection.

| 1981
The Feline Virus Unit established under the directorship of Os Jarrett.

63

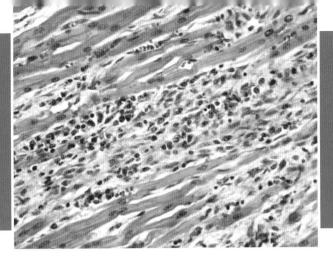

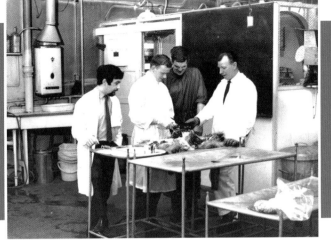

Parvovirus myocarditis   *Norman Wright and Hal Thompson in post mortem room, Buccleuch Street*

Unravelling the cause of kennel cough

In the late 1970s the group then began work that helped unravel the aetiology of the perplexing condition of infectious canine tracheobronchitis (kennel cough). Emphasis on research on canine respiratory disease had become concentrated on viruses: CDV, CAV-1, a second type of canine adenovirus (CAV-2) discovered in 1961 in Canada, and canine parainfluenza virus (CPIV) uncovered in 1976 by the Glasgow group.

Bordetella bronchiseptica had long been known to occur in dogs with respiratory disease, often associated with CDV, but had been somewhat neglected as the emphasis had turned to viruses. The group therefore set out to reassess the role of Bordetella in kennel cough. In experimental infections they showed that *B. bronchiseptica* was a primary pathogen. They then went on to define the pathology of the condition in field cases from which they attempted to isolate possible aetiological agents.

It was concluded that *B. bronchiseptica* and CPIV were the most significant pathogens and that neither CDV nor CAV were the prime causes. These conclusions have been confirmed extensively throughout the world.

The pandemic of canine parvovirus

A novel virus, canine parvovirus (CPV), emerged in 1979 with devastating consequences for dogs. The Glasgow group were in the forefront of its discovery. That year Hal Thompson and colleagues described outbreaks of sudden death due to myocarditis in puppies in the west of Scotland and in England. They found inclusions in the nuclei of cardiac myocytes and proposed a virus as a cause. Later that year they isolated a parvovirus from older dogs with enteritis and suggested that the two syndromes were different manifestations of infection by the same virus. Subsequently Lawson Macartney and colleagues carried out a large series of experimental infections that defined the pathogenesis of these conditions and developed methods for diagnosis and control.

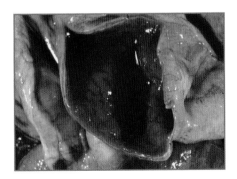

Gut affected by parvovirus

Diagnostic serology for canine viruses

The serological expertise of the group was called upon in the 1998 epidemic of fatal disease in harbour seals in the Scottish waters of the North Sea caused by phocine distemper virus. Using tests for antibody developed for the related CDV, Campbell Cornwell and colleagues from the University of Aberdeen showed that grey seals first came into contact with the virus at the time of the epidemic but survived, indicating that grey seals were much less susceptible to the virus than harbour seals.

One of the most significant practical contributions of the group to dog welfare was testing the efficacy of canine viral vaccines in the field. Precise serological tests were developed which could be used to correlate antibody levels in vaccinated dogs with protection from challenge. In collaborations with veterinary practitioners throughout the UK, serum samples were obtained from thousands of pups being vaccinated with commercial vaccines. The results facilitated the selection of the safest and most effective vaccines and the elimination of the worst; and contributed to the acceptance of vaccination schedules that ensured protection of the vast majority of vaccinated pups.

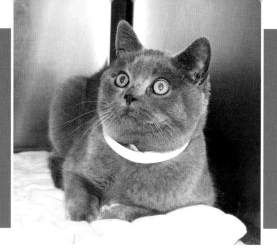
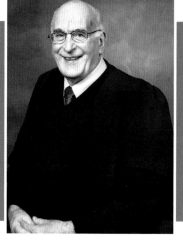
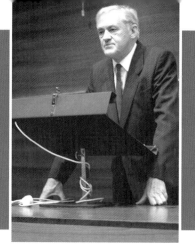

Feline virology

In 1961 Bill Jarrett obtained funding from the British Empire Cancer Campaign (now Cancer Research UK) to investigate with Bill Martin the cause of leukaemia in domestic animals. Michael Stoker provided laboratory space at the newly built Institute of Virology for Bill Martin and his research technologist colleague David Hay, who had worked in Kenya with the eminent veterinary virologist Walter Plowright, to carry out the virology part of the work. Their extensive study on bovine lymphoma in the UK showed that the form of the disease most prevalent in continental Europe and North America, enzootic bovine leukosis, which was shown subsequently in the USA to be caused by bovine leukaemia virus, did not occur in the UK; hence it was not surprising in retrospect that they did not isolate a virus from local cases.

Discovery of feline leukaemia virus

By contrast, their virology work on cat lymphoma was spectacularly successful and the cause, feline leukaemia virus (FeLV), was discovered. Bill Jarrett's attention was drawn by local practitioner Harry Pfaff to a cluster of cases of lymphoma that occurred over a short period of time in cats in the house of one of his clients.

Bill's belief that this was caused by an infectious agent was confirmed by reproducing the disease in transmission experiments and finding a retrovirus in the resulting tumours, which resembled the viruses then known to cause leukaemia in laboratory mice and domestic poultry. The pathological and transmission studies were carried out at the Veterinary School at Garscube and the cell culture and electron microscopy studies, by which the virus was first visualised, were done at the Institute of Virology.

The discovery of FeLV in 1964 was an important event in veterinary and comparative medicine. It added to the realisation at the time that viruses might be important causes of cancers in man and provided one of the major justifications for an application to the US Congress for massive research support to set up the Special Virus Cancer Program that ran from 1968 until 1980.

Although the initial search for viruses in human cancers was disappointing, Bill Jarrett's finding that FeLV caused mainly lymphomas of T-cell origin in the cat persuaded Robert Gallo to persist with virus hunting and led ultimately to the latter's discovery of the human T-cell leukaemia virus, HTLV, in the early 1980s and subsequently his co-discovery of human immunodeficiency virus (HIV).

Defining the natural history of FeLV

At the School, the discovery of FeLV gave access to a major funding source from the cancer research charities, which supported a large group investigating the pathogenesis and epidemiology of the virus and subsequently devising methods to diagnose and control the infection. This work spawned other research areas such as molecular oncology and the establishment of the Human Virus Centre by the Leukaemia Research Fund (now Leukaemia and Lymphoma UK). Following the discovery of FeLV, funding was obtained to extend virology research at Garscube. New recruits included Bill Jarrett's brother Oswald (Os), who had just finished his PhD studies at the Institute of Virology in 1965, pathologist Lindsay Mackey and Helen Laird, an electron microscopist from the University of Strathclyde.

A small wooden building was converted into a laboratory (known rather grandiosely as the 'Pfizer Building' as it had been provided by a grant from the Pfizer pharmaceutical company for research on coccidiosis in poultry but was never occupied by chickens) and was equipped with an electron microscope and a cell culture suite. This new, tiny laboratory became the focus for a large network of research on FeLV that was established in Europe and the USA.

1983

Tom Douglas becomes Dean.

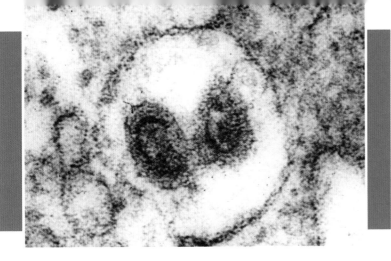

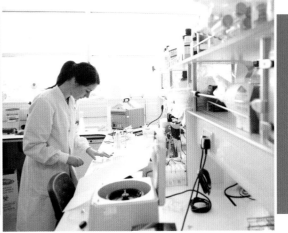

Diagnostic methods were developed which were used in field and experimental studies by Os Jarrett, David Hay and Matt Golder to define the interaction of the virus and its host. Cats exposed to the virus either became persistently viraemic or mounted an immune response and recovered. Subsequently Angela Pacitti found that in many ostensibly recovered cats a latent infection lingered on for several years, although without causing any apparent harm. The infection was found to be common and in some multicat households prevalence reached forty percent. However, by separating viraemic cats from non-viraemic animals it was possible to prevent further spread of the virus.

A diagnostic service was offered to veterinary practitioners in the UK who enthusiastically applied it to eliminate the infection, particularly in pedigree cats. In subsequent years, with the production of rapid, in-practice tests and the development of vaccines, the prevalence of FeLV infection has been reduced to such an extent that it is now uncommon in British cats.

It soon became clear that FeLV was associated with several different types of cancer and cytopaenias in cats and the question arose whether each was caused by a distinct virus type. Isolates from the field were found to belong to three main subgroups, A, B or C of which A was present in all isolates, B was found in addition to A in about half, while C, again together with A, was rare. In fact, FeLV-A is the common form that is transmitted between cats and the other subgroups arise *in vivo* by modifications of the envelope gene of this virus.

Transmission studies found that A and B caused lymphoma while C caused a very specific, fatal anaemia. Detailed analysis of this latter condition by David Onions and collaborators at the Paterson Laboratory in Manchester, pinpointed the defect in erythropoiesis in infected cats. Searching for the reason why this disease is specific to FeLV-C, a haematology research group in Seattle working with Brian Willett identified the cell receptor for FeLV-C as a haem transporter molecule and explained the pathogenesis of the anaemia at the molecular level. Further analysis found that mutations in the human equivalent of the receptor are responsible for Blackfan Diamond anaemia in children and a lethal vascular disorder of the human foetus, Fowler Syndrome.

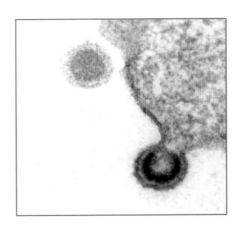

Electron micrograph of retrovirus

The molecular biology of FeLV

In 1980 Jim Neil, who had completed his PhD studies in Os Jarrett's laboratory, returned to Glasgow after spending three years as a postdoctoral fellow at the University of Southern California. On joining the Beatson Institute for Cancer Research at Garscube, he set up an extremely valuable collaboration between his group and the FeLV laboratory at the School. Bringing his molecular biology experience to the subject he uncovered the molecular basis of lymphoma development in FeLV-infected cats, where the virus activates cellular oncogenes by several distinct mechanisms. His group, including long-term associates Monica Stewart and Anne Terry, established the origin of FeLV-B as a recombinant between the infectious FeLV-A and endogenous FeLV envelope genes. In addition, Mark Rigby showed how a mutation in the env gene of FeLV-A produces FeLV-C which causes erythroid aplasia. Another key achievement from the Beatson-Vet School collaboration was the molecular cloning of the FeLV-A Glasgow-1 strain, leading to the generation of a recombinant vaccine for FeLV in collaboration with Merial. This very effective vaccine that includes the structural genes of the Glasgow strain in a canary pox virus vector is now available worldwide as *Purevax FeLV*. This represented the first commercial use of a live vectored vaccine against a retroviral disease.

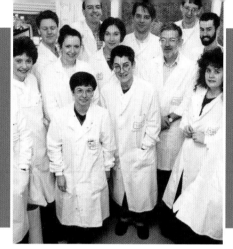
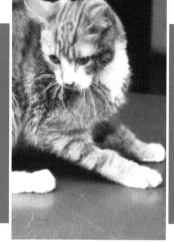
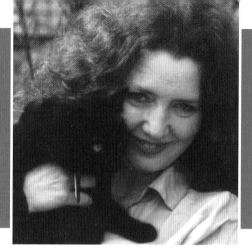

MRC Retrovirus Research group 1990   A cat infected with FIP   Diane Addie

Feline immunodeficiency virus as a model for AIDS

In 1987 the MRC established the AIDS Directed Programme with the aim of producing vaccines and antivirals to control HIV. Bill Jarrett was one of the founding members and together with Jim Neil and Os Jarrett was awarded a programme grant to develop feline immunodeficiency virus (FIV), which had recently been discovered in California, as a vaccine model for HIV. To facilitate this work while continuing to pursue his molecular oncology interests, Jim transferred his Beatson Institute group to newly refurbished laboratories in the School in 1992.

A serological survey in the UK by Margaret Hosie revealed that FIV was a common infection in cats, affecting about five percent overall. FIV was found not to be as lethal as FeLV in experimental cats but did produce significant morbidity of cats in the field. The pathogenesis of experimental infection was studied by Sean Callanan and Christine Lawrence, antibody responses by Bob Osborne and cellular immunity by Julia Beatty and Norman Flynn. Several vaccines were tested with immunogens ranging from inactivated virus, through recombinant proteins to molecularly cloned FIV DNA. Significant humoral and cellular immune responses to the virus were induced and protection from challenge was achieved, but only to FIV strains that had been attenuated by growth in cell culture and not to a representative local virulent isolate.

Alarmingly, enhancement of infection by some vaccines was evident, which was a dramatic warning for the development of vaccines for HIV. It was also found by Stephen Dunham that the commercial FIV vaccine that had been produced in the USA did not protect against infection by the non-attenuated strain, which reinforced the evidence for the refusal by the authorities of a license to market the vaccine in the UK. Research on the reasons for the differences in virulence of FIV strains by Brian Willett and Margaret Hosie led to characterisation of the crucial mechanisms by which the virus enters cells and, with Japanese colleagues, identification of the cell surface receptors utilised by FIV. They continue to explore the basics of FIV biology which may influence the production of effective vaccines.

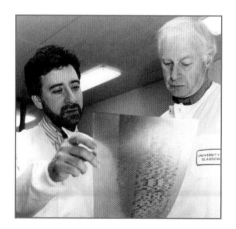

First sequence of FIV; Jim Neil and Os Jarrett

Feline infectious peritonitis

In the Feline Virus Unit, research was also conducted on aspects of other common feline viruses including feline calicivirus and feline herpesvirus, but particularly on feline coronavirus (FCoV), the cause of feline infectious peritonitis (FIP), by Diane Addie. FIP is now the most important infectious diseases of cats in the UK. Her innovative work in the field, following up FCoV infections in more than 800 cats and 400 kittens over periods of three to twelve years, revealed that FIP occurred mainly as an uncommon outcome following the first infection of young cats with FCoV.

Using the same resource, she and Lesley Nicolson explored the molecular epidemiology of FCoV and showed that the factors that influence whether FCoV establishes lifelong infection in some cats and not others are determined mainly by the host response to infection.

With Susan Duthie and David Eckersall, she developed very useful diagnostic aids for FIP, which had been previously a difficult condition to diagnose. She also established methods to control FCoV infection which have been successfully implemented in many multicat households.

1986

James Armour becomes Dean.

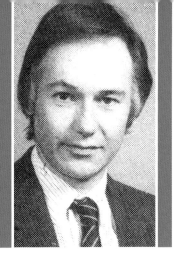

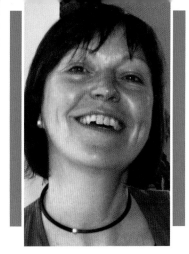

One of the most successful spin-out companies to emerge from Glasgow University was created within the Faculty, prior to the existence of the incubator facilities. Q-One Biotech Limited was founded in 1990 on Kelvin Campus with just five employees, based on the work of Professor David Onions, and became a world-renowned company providing specialist safety testing services,

cGMP contract manufacturing of cell banks and gene therapy products and virus validation services to the biopharmaceutical industry. In 1994 it transferred to a larger facility on Todd Campus. By the time the company was sold in 2003 for £42M to BioReliance Corporation it had expanded to more than 170 employees.

David Onions   *Ruth Jarrett*

Molecular oncology

The move of Jim Neil's group from the Beatson Institute in 1992 was secured by the establishment of the Molecular Oncology Laboratory in collaboration with David Onions and his former PhD student Ewan Cameron. David left to lead his highly successful start-up company Q-One Biotech on a full-time basis in 1996. The Molecular Oncology Laboratory forms a group of around a dozen scientists that has been funded by a unique joint programme grant from Cancer Research UK and Leukaemia & Lymphoma Research. Following the leads from cellular oncogenes discovered in the study of FeLV, they established new mouse models of haematopoietic cancer, taking advantage of the advances in transgenic technology and the completion of the mouse genome sequence in 2001. Among their notable achievements is the use of insertional mutagenesis to identify a family of transcription factors, the Runx genes, as important targets in cancer, attracting further international collaborations and interest in the School's research activities.

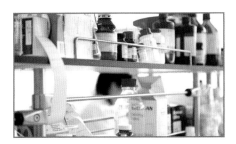

The Leukaemia Research Fund Virus Centre

The Leukaemia Research Fund (LRF) Virus Centre was established in 1986 to study viruses as causative agents of human leukaemia and lymphoma. The Virus Centre was located at the School because of the Pathology Department's longstanding interest and expertise in animal leukaemia viruses and virus discovery. David Onions was the first director, followed by Ruth Jarrett in 1991. The Centre is housed in purpose-built laboratories within the Ian Botham Building.

The group investigates the role of viruses in human leukaemia and lymphoma with a particular focus on virus discovery. Early efforts concentrated on culturing a broad range of leukaemia and lymphoma samples for evidence of viral infection, largely using electron microscopy. Subsequently, research focused on the study of Hodgkin lymphoma and childhood leukaemia, two diseases where the epidemiology suggested involvement of an infectious agent. Both are associated with a high standard of living and some degree of social isolation in early childhood leading to the idea that delayed infection with a common infectious agent could play a role in disease pathogenesis.

The group were involved in showing that the Epstein-Barr virus (EBV) is causatively involved in some cases of Hodgkin lymphoma. This is a ubiquitous herpes virus that causes infectious mononucleosis (glandular fever) and is associated with lymphoproliferative disease in immunosuppressed persons. Around one-third of cases in the UK are associated with EBV and work at the Virus Centre showed that EBV-associated and non-associated Hodgkin lymphoma cases have distinct demographic features and risk factors. This led the group to propose the four-disease model of classical Hodgkin lymphoma, which divides the disease into four groups of cases on the basis of EBV association, age at diagnosis and age of infection with EBV. Recent international collaborative studies investigating the role of host genetics in disease risk support the idea that EBV-associated and non-associated cases have a distinct pathogenesis and show that polymorphisms in Human Leukocyte Antigen genes play a key role in determining disease risk. The group has continued to pursue the search for a virus in EBV-negative Hodgkin lymphoma cases. Early studies involved attempts to culture the tumour cells but during the late 1990s the emphasis changed to molecular methods of virus discovery. In recent years, the advent of massively parallel sequencing using 'Next Generation Sequencing' methods has revolutionised virus discovery techniques. Although the techniques are still new and the bioinformatic challenge is daunting, it is hoped that any directly transforming agent, present in the tumour cells in Hodgkin lymphoma, will be unearthed.

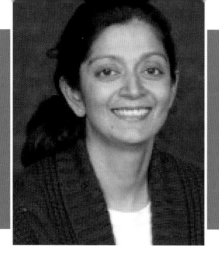
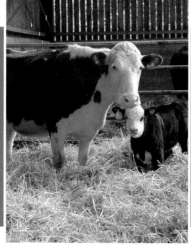
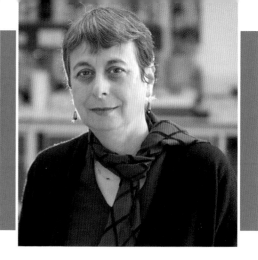

Lubna Nasir

Saveria Campo

Bovine viral diseases

Skin diseases

During his time in East Africa, Bill Martin with Myrtle Pirie and Maureen Flannigan had investigated pseudo-lumpy-skin disease caused by Allerton virus, now known as bovine herpesvirus type 2. Back at the Veterinary School in Glasgow in 1966, following his work on FeLV, he discovered with Ian Lauder and local practitioner Brian Martin an identical virus as the cause of ulcerative mammillitis in dairy cattle in the west of Scotland.

Further studies during the subsequent five years defined the clinical, pathological and virological features of this and other similar skin conditions of cattle, including cowpox, pseudocowpox and papillomas and provided useful parameters for differential diagnosis.

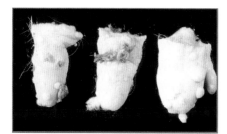

Teat of bovine mammary gland demonstrating viral wart

Bovine papillomaviruses

Bill Jarrett and his colleagues also worked on bovine papillomavirus (BPV), 'one of his favourite virus groups, those causing the humble wart, verruca and angleberry'. New techniques in molecular biology had shown that humans and cattle had several papilloma viruses, each usually associated with a particular disease. In the 1970s and 1980s, following his observations in the 1960s of papillomas in association with clusters of vulvo-cutaneous carcinomas in Friesian cattle in the Highlands of Kenya, he investigated, with Pauline McNeil and clinical colleagues Ian Selman, Bill Grimshaw and Ian McIntyre, the reasons for a high incidence of alimentary tract carcinoma in cattle in parts of upland Scotland and the north of England. He discovered a new virus, BPV-4, in frond papillomas of the upper alimentary tract of cattle, and found that this virus caused cancer in association with the consumption of bracken, which is known to contain chemical carcinogens. His discovery was the definitive proof that papillomaviruses are indeed implicated in cancer development.

In this and subsequent studies he collaborated closely with Saveria Campo and her molecular biology group at the Beatson Institute. They made further discoveries, including a new BPV subgroup, BPV-6, that causes a true epithelial papilloma of the mammary gland skin.

In the 1990s after a thorough study of the biology of the known bovine papillomaviruses, they developed recombinant protein vaccines for BPV-4, one of which (L2) protected calves against challenge with the virus and one (E7) which, remarkably, was therapeutic, inducing rejection of existing carcinomas. The former prototype vaccine showed the feasibility of vaccine protection and served as the direct forerunner of the recently introduced vaccine for cervical cancer in women caused by human papillomaviruses.

Supported by a Cancer Research UK Life Fellowship, Saveria relocated from the Beatson Institute to the Veterinary School in 1999 to continue to work on the comparative medicine theme, studying bovine and human papillomaviruses in collaboration with colleagues including Iain Morgan, Lubna Nasir and Sheila Graham. Even after Saveria's retirement, Glasgow continued to host one of the largest groups of papillomavirus researchers in the UK. Their recent interests have included the mechanisms by which papillomaviruses evade host immune responses and overcome barriers to replication, potentially sensitive points in the viral lifecycle that may be amenable to novel interventions in virus-infected individuals.

1987

Ian Botham opens the Leukaemia Research Fund Virus Centre.

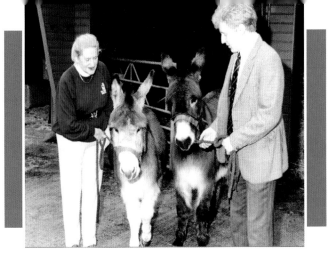

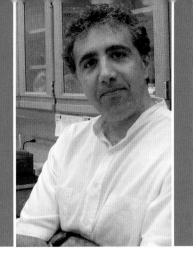

Massimo Palmarini is a veterinary graduate of the University of Perugia. He completed his PhD studies at the Moredun Research Institute then worked at Stanford and the College of Veterinary Medicine of the University of Georgia before being appointed to a newly established chair in Molecular Pathogenesis in the Faculty of Veterinary Medicine in Glasgow.

Elisabeth Svendsen with Stuart Reid

Equine sarcoid

In 1991, Stuart Reid and Bill Jarrett discovered in donkeys that a papillomavirus was the causative agent of sarcoid, a common skin tumour in equines. The work was funded by Dr Elisabeth Svendsen's Donkey Sanctuary. Stuart Reid, Lubna Nasir and Saveria Campo demonstrated that bovine papilloma viruses type 1 and 2 were involved. Lubna continued this research and with the close cooperation of Saveria secured grant funding for numerous projects ranging from evolutionary studies of the worldwide distribution of BPV variants in equids and bovids, to investigations of viral pathogenesis and interactions of the virus with host cell defences.

The most significant findings included the demonstration that equine sarcoids are associated with BPV sequence variants that differ from isolates found in cattle, implying that the infection is transmitted from horse to horse and does not arise from cattle, as was previously believed. The group also found that flies may act as mechanical vectors for disease transmission. An exciting recent discovery is that sarcoids can regress following therapy with a genetically modified vaccine in both horses and donkeys.

Bridging human and animal virology

From 1961 the Institute of Virology was based in new laboratories on Church Street, and served as a major UK centre for basic research on viruses. In 2009 the MRC decided to terminate its funding and invited tenders from academic institutions throughout the UK to host a new unit for experimental virus research. A bid from the University of Glasgow, championed by Jim Neil, was successful following major international reviews and intense competition from across the UK. An award of £28M was made to establish the Centre for Virus Research (CVR), including £6M to support a new building on the School campus at Garscube.

In 2010, Massimo Palmarini was appointed as the first Director of the CVR. Massimo conducts basic research on Jaagsiekte sheep retrovirus which he has shown formally was the cause of ovine pulmonary adenocarcinoma, a common tumour of sheep; and that a structural protein of the virus directly transformed type II pneumocytes to cancer cells. In addition, he has demonstrated that endogenous forms of the virus are used by sheep to regulate peri-implantation placental growth and differentiation in the embryo.

The occurrence of these viruses in different breeds of sheep has also been exploited to provide valuable insights into the history of sheep domestication. Recently his group has begun a programme to understand the determinants of bluetongue virus (BTV) pathogenesis and to understand the main factors that control the clinical outcome of BTV infection in ruminants, which can be variable. The aim is to design control strategies that fit the risks posed by a specific BTV outbreak.

The CVR comprises a unique international research centre with around 200 staff dedicated to the study of human and animal viral diseases. The mission of the CVR is to carry out multidisciplinary research on viruses and viral diseases of humans and animals, translating the knowledge gained for the improvement of human and animal health. The new CVR building will be linked to the Henry Wellcome Building for Comparative Medical Sciences, and is due to be operational by 2014.

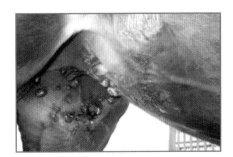

Equine sarcoid

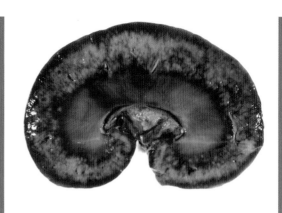

Acute interstitial nephtitis, leptospirosis

Bacteriology

Stanislaw Michna was the major figure in Bacteriology from the 1950s to 1972. Originally from Poland, he had a qualification in bacteriology from the University of Lvov and was in the Polish Army Veterinary Corps on the Eastern Front at the outbreak of World War II. The fact that most of his colleagues who surrendered to the Russians were subsequently massacred at Katyn remained an enduring influence on his attitudes to the post-war Eastern Bloc governments. After a hair-raising escape from occupied Europe during the War, he re-qualified as MRCVS at Edinburgh and moved to Glasgow where he taught bacteriology and some virology to undergraduates, by whom he was remembered as a strong and somewhat idiosyncratic character. He carried out diagnostic serology, particularly for leptospirosis and brucellosis, worked closely with medical bacteriologists in Glasgow on the human aspects of these diseases and carried out ground-breaking research into leptospirosis. The work he conducted on brucellosis with the medical bacteriologists was of particular relevance to the student body, over 60 percent of whom seroconverted to brucellosis during the Glasgow course in the late 1960s. This seems unbelievable today, but the disease was widespread at a time when rubber gloves and proper protective clothing were not readily available.

Part of his success with leptospiral culture was due to his meticulous preparation of reagents and his rigorous selection of specimens. This feature of his work was not always popular with the technical staff involved, but it allowed him to isolate organisms from animals with a success rate that no one else in the UK could match. He worked extensively with canine leptospirosis, isolating the agents responsible and providing a comprehensive serological diagnostic service. He also explored the pathogenicity of the then *L. canicola* for pigs. However, he made his most lasting contribution researching ruminant leptospirosis. He found antibodies to a wide variety of leptospiral serogroups in cattle and explored the relationships between cattle and wildlife, culminating in the identification of the then *L. hardjo* as the cause of many bovine abortions, and the discovery that cattle were its maintenance host. This was confirmed experimentally with his final research student, Bill Ellis, and the knowledge gained allowed him to devise eradication programmes for infected cattle. During a two year post-retirement BBSRC fellowship, he produced and tested a vaccine from his isolate together with Burroughs Wellcome.

Maurice Grindlay worked in bacteriology from the 1960s until his early retirement in the early 1980s. He and his technician Douglas Ramsay, were responsible for the routine bacteriology diagnostic work generated by the veterinary school and contributed to the teaching.

Maurice was colour blind - a real problem for a classic bacteriologist - and had to rely on Douglas to interpret the Ziehl Nielsen stains for him, although he could manage to distinguish Gram stains in shades of grey. His particular interests were in the role of *E. coli* in canine cystitis and in canine pyometra, then a serious and often fatal canine condition.

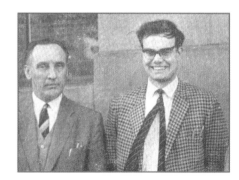

Stanislaw Michna and Ronald Roberts 1960s

1988
Sir James Black, is awarded the Nobel Prize in Physiology and Medicine.

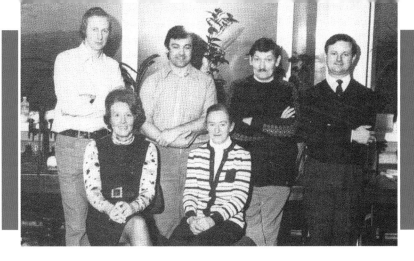
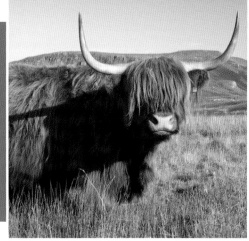

Oswald Jarrett, David Taylor, Maurice Grindlay, Campbell Cornwell, Christine Dawson and Helen Laird 1970s

David Taylor arrived from Cambridge in 1972 as a replacement for Stanislaw Michna and carried on the latter's diagnostic and survey work with leptospira until the Great Fire of 1982, when the microbiology laboratories were gutted. Bacteriology was only damaged by water and pasteurised by the heat, but had to decamp to portacabins for 18 months until the repairs were complete. His main areas of research were the bacterial diseases of farm livestock, especially pigs, and for twenty five years he carried out pathogenicity studies on pigs and trials of new therapies on pig antimicrobials in converted Nissen huts at Cochno. Notable discoveries included the reproduction in 1980 of spirochaetal diarrhoea or porcine colonic spirochaetosis with the first isolate (made the type species in 1995) of *Brachyspira pilosicoli*, now one of the most commonly diagnosed enteric diseases of pigs in the UK. Research topics in pigs included enteric diseases, respiratory diseases, especially pleuropneumonia which he conducted either alone or with Andrew Rycroft, and studies of pig disease in the field which led to the publication of the book 'Pig Diseases'.

Work on cattle included surveys of the bacteria present in enteric lesions and the reproduction of campylobacter infections, most notably *Campylobacter jejuni* infection, and clostridial infections.

Chris Dawson provided mycological expertise from the 1960s until her retirement in the early 1980s. Her early work involved the evaluation of Griseofulvin as a treatment for ringworm in animals. Later, with colleagues in the department of Veterinary Medicine, she studied the role of agricultural fungal antigens in disease, especially in farmer's lung, and subsequnetly in aspergillosis in dogs and horses.

Andrew Rycroft replaced Maurice Grindlay and studied *Actinobacillus pleuropneumoniae*, the cause of porcine pleuropneumonia, describing Apx III for the first time and defining the toxins produced by the different serotypes of the organism. He moved on the Royal Veterinary College in the late 1990s.

Mark Roberts succeeded Dr Rycroft. His group has defined virulence factors in *Actinobacillus pleuropneumoniae* and *Salmonella enterica serovar Typhimurium*, and on the detection of carriers of *E. coli* O157 in cattle. Dr Paul Everest joined the laboratory in the late 1990s and concentrated on pathogenic mechanisms in *Campylobacter jejuni*, using the pig as an experimental model and adopting genetic manipulation techniques to study its genetic basis.

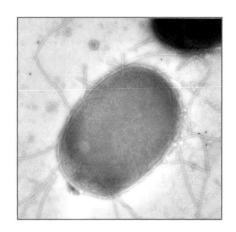

Salmonella

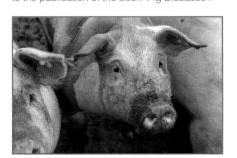

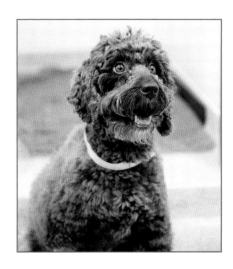

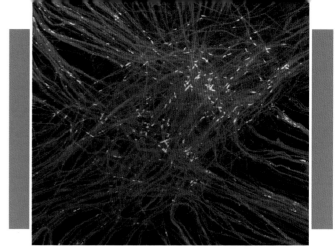

Myelinating culture; axons ensheathed in myelin, with nodes of Ranvier (green).

Neuroscience

The Wellcome Surgical Institute

With the relocation of the Veterinary School to the Garscube campus, three far-sighted individuals, William Weipers, Arthur MacKay, St Mungo Professor of Surgery at the Royal Infirmary, and Sir Charles Illingworth, Regius Professor of Surgery at the Western Infirmary, recognised the importance of the two principles which still guide biomedical research today: the creation of a dynamic research environment, and the promotion of interactions between basic animal research and clinical practice, so-called translational research. They received funding from The Wellcome Trust to build a translational medicine institute which was opened in October 1960 by Sir Henry Dale, a Nobel Laureate.

The mission of the Wellcome Surgical Institute, as it eventually became, was 'to provide facilities for members of the medical and veterinary schools of the University of Glasgow to enable them to carry out research into problems in the broad field of medical sciences relating to diseases of man and animals or investigation of fundamental factors which may be important in causing disease'. The first steward was Murray Harper who was pivotal in setting the ethos of the Institute and guiding its expansion.

Over fifty years, the Institute made seminal advances in many areas of medicine which include: the development in animals of methods for measuring brain blood flow in man using radioactive inert gases (featured in the iconic BBC series 'Tomorrow's World' in the late 1960s); defining the contribution of axons and oligodendrocytes to acute and chronic damage to white matter in animals and man (Ian Griffiths); insight gained into the aetiology of hypertension (by the MRC Blood Pressure Unit at the Western Infirmary led by Tony Lever); elucidating how cerebral blood flow was regulated in health and disease (the MRC Cerebral Circulation Group led by Bryan Jennett and Murray Harper); the development by James McCulloch, together with his neurosurgical colleagues from around the globe, of the first model of focal cerebral ischaemia (stroke) in rodents, a model which has underpinned research in this area for twentyfive years; and the refinement of cardiac bypass and the development of new cardiac surgical techniques (by David Wheatley and his colleagues).

The success of the Institute was recognised by repeated expansion and by acquisition of major competitive rewards, from the first programme grant from The Wellcome Trust in 1977 (a joint application from veterinary surgeons, neurosurgeons and basic scientists) to the award in 2002 from the Scottish Executive to establish 7. Tesla magnetic resonance imaging (MRI) at Garscube (another joint bid from vets, human clinicians and basic scientists).

In the first Research Assessment Exercise in 1986, the Wellcome Surgical Institute had the rare distinction of being awarded the highest grade of 'outstanding'. The Institute continues to fulfil its original mission within the College of Medical, Veterinary and Life Sciences whose creation was to foster interdisciplinary research collaboration, the same goals of the visionaries who created the Institute over fifty years ago.

1991

Norman Wright becomes Dean.

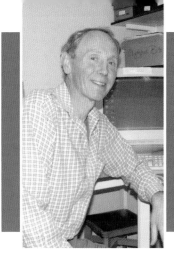

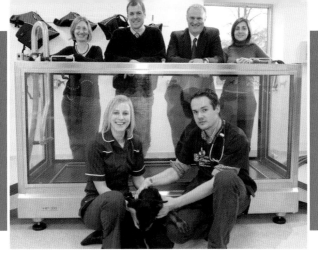

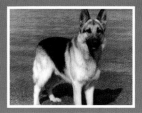

Ian Griffiths | Neurology team 2012 | Rebel Hodges

Neurology

Neurology at the School began with Donald Lawson who adapted simple physiological tests, such as spinal reflexes, for use in the clinics. This, together with radiology, allowed fairly accurate localisation of spinal cord lesions. Myelography was also employed although the agents available were inefficient and dangerous compared with modern contrast media. Similar adaptation of experimental physiological findings allowed some localisation of brain lesions.

Another twentyfive to thirty years would pass before computed tomography and MRI became available and affordable for veterinary neurology. In 1968 Ian Griffiths was appointed as a lecturer with special interest in neurology. He adapted the small histology laboratory in the Surgery Department to specialise in neuropathology, developing contacts with the relevant medical departments and the Wellcome Surgical Institute. This allowed detailed pathological examinations to be correlated with clinical findings.

The early work concentrated on spinal cord damage, particularly due to intervertebral disc problems, and the role of impaired blood flow. One of the early successes was the first description of fibrocartilagenous emboli as a cause of cord infarction, now recognised as a common problem.

In the early 1970s a purpose-built electromyography machine was acquired which allowed detailed electrophysiological studies of nerve and muscle lesions to be performed on clinical cases. Ian Duncan, now Professor of Neurology at Wisconsin USA, joined the unit to study idiopathic laryngeal hemiplegia (roaring) in the horse. The lab was extended to handle specialised peripheral nerve and muscle samples, and electron microscopy was introduced. Several new diseases were recognised and characterised, such as giant axonal neuropathy in German Shepherds, sensory neuropathy in Long Haired Dachshunds, progressive axonopathy in Boxers, and congenital myotonia in Chows.

In the early 1980s a new feline disorder appeared throughout the UK and was identified clinically and pathologically by the neurologists at Glasgow as a dysautonomia with remarkable similarities to equine grass sickness. Similar dysautonomias were subsequently recognised in dogs and hares. Through the 1980s and early 1990s the range of investigations applicable to biopsy and post mortem tissue expanded to include immunocytochemical and molecular techniques.

The emphasis of the research work also shifted from peripheral nerve to disorders of myelin and the interactions between axons and the myelin sheaths in the central nervous system. The discovery in 1981 of dogs with a mutation in the major myelin protein *Plp* gene (shaking pup) was followed by identification of rodents with mutations in the same gene. These mutant animals proved valid models for a rare human disorder, Pelizaeus-Merzbacher disease and also provided insights into the role of myelin in maintaining axonal integrity, factors that are relevant to multiple sclerosis. This line of work led to fruitful collaboration with other groups in the UK, USA and Germany and the application of powerful tools in mouse genetics to study these topics.

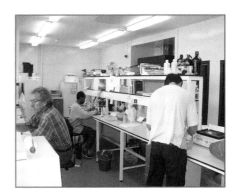

Neurology laboratory

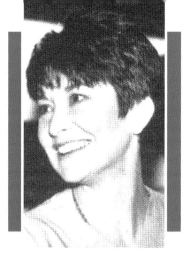

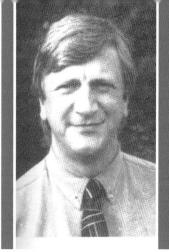

Neil Gorman

Professor Neil Gorman, a graduate of the Universities of Liverpool and Cambridge, was appointed as Professor of Surgery in 1986 in time to become involved in the Riley review on the future of the Glasgow Veterinary School.

During his tenure he encouraged new young blood into the department, *in particular to strengthen its research profile and also to redevelop and update small animal surgery. While at Glasgow, equine surgery eventually moved to the new equine facility. In 1993, he joined Mars Incorporated. Neil became Vice-Chancellor of Nottingham Trent University in 2003. He was President of the RCVS during 1997-98 and received an honorary DVMS from the University of Glasgow in 2004.*

Jacqueline Reid   Neil Gorman

Pain research

Research into the management of pain in animals began in Glasgow with work undertaken by Andrea Nolan and Jacqueline Reid in the early 1990s. At that time the extent of pain in animals could not readily be assessed and consequently the management of pain was very patchy: many veterinary surgeons did not use analgesic drugs in routine surgical procedures in companion animals, and pain management in farm animals was confined primarily to the use of local anaesthetics for the performance of surgery. Their early work was in the use of peri-operative analgesics drugs to manage acute pain, the outcomes of which successfully contributed to the more routine use of analgesics drugs.

This work also led to the development of new infusion protocols for total intravenous anaesthesia, supplemented by the delivery of low dose analgesics through target controlled infusions.

Later they teamed up with statistician Marian Scott and began a long-term collaboration evaluating simple pain scales commonly used in humans. Having assessed the use of the scales in dogs, they developed and validated the Glasgow Composite Pain Scale (GCPS) for the assessment of acute pain in dogs, the first interval-level scale for use in any animal species.

Thereafter they produced a shortened version, the GCPS- SF, a tool that is now recommended in a variety of veterinary textbooks and is freely available for download and use. The group expanded to draw in Lesley Wiseman-Orr and together they developed a tool for chronic pain in dogs, focussing on the impact of chronic pain on animal quality of life. This has been developed for use by owners, is now available in a web-based format and has been validated in dogs with a range of chronic conditions. The group expanded their work to farm animals, collaborating with Julie Fitzpatrick on cattle and sheep. This research complemented Andrea's work on the spinal neurobiology of clinical pain in foot rot and mastitis, work she carried out with Sharron Dolan and others in a collaboration that began in the mid 1990s and continues.

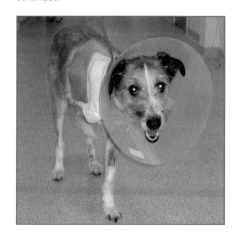

Orthopaedic research

The School has consistently made a major contribution to orthopaedic research. In the 1950s Donald Lawson popularised the technique of Rush-pinning for fractures of the distal femur in dogs and cats, a technique which he adapted from human orthopaedic surgery. This was at a time when internal fixation of fractures in veterinary patients was very much in its infancy.

He also made a very significant contribution to the radiological diagnosis of canine hip dysplasia in the early 1960s which formed the basis of the British Veterinary Association/ Kennel Club scoring scheme for this disease. His colleague and friend Jimmy Campbell was one of the early pioneers in research into the nutritional bone diseases in growing dogs which were common in the 1950s and 1960s when commercial diets were less readily available and owners tended to feed diets low in calcium and high in phosphorous to their pets resulting in osteopaenia.

In the early 1970s the appointment of Melvyn Pond to the Surgery department heralded the beginning of a long period of a very significant research into arthritic diseases of the dog and cat, much of it having very important comparative relevance.

1995
James Armour receives knighthood.

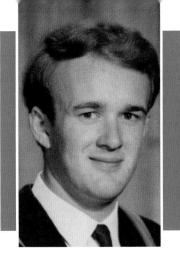
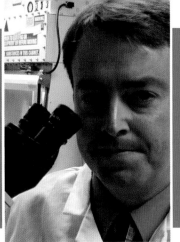
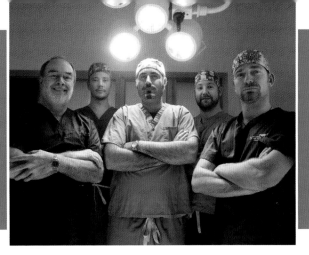

Melvyn Pond   *David Argyle*   *Orthopaedic team 2010*

Melvyn worked with George Nuki, the Professor of Rheumatology in the Medical Faculty and established the cruciate sectioning model of osteoarthritis in the dog, the so-called Pond-Nuki model. In collaboration with the Kennedy Institute in London studies were carried out on the degenerative processes affecting articular cartilage in osteoarthritis. Liz White (nee Gilbertson) was another member of this group whose work on osteophyte development in osteoarthritis was a seminal study which challenged the idea that osteophyte development was a relatively late manifestation of the pathology that followed the cartilage changes.

Following the departure of Melvyn Pond to the USA, David Bennett was appointed as Lecturer in Surgery. He continued to forge links with the Medical School in Glasgow, particularly with the rheumatology department. This led to the identification of a number of previously unrecognised rheumatic diseases in small animals, including rheumatoid arthritis which was previously only thought to affect humans. David's collaboration with Bill Ollier and his group (the Mammalian Immunogenetics Research Group based at the Universities of Liverpool and Manchester) showed a genetic susceptibility to canine rheumatoid arthritis that was very similar to that for the human.

Following David's return to Glasgow, later research into arthritis with David Argyle and Lubna Nasir using tissue culture techniques described the potential of gene therapy to control osteoarthritis.

Sarah Campbell demonstrated that genes to inhibit inflammatory cytokines and the matrix metalloproteinases which destroy articular cartilage in osteoarthritis can be inserted into chondrocytes and synovial cells to slow down the degenerative process. What was more intriguing was that the therapeutic genes could be controlled by gene promoters which were activated by the disease process itself, and by promoters which were specific to certain cell types such as chondrocytes.

Thus a targeted, self-regulating gene therapy system was created; the group aims to use the system in clinical cases. More recently the group has been studying the role of cartilage senescence in the osteoarthritic disease process.

The studies have also shown that oxidative stress, a well known by-product of joint inflammation is a strong inducer of senescence. Reversal of cartilage senescence by, for example, telomerase gene therapy or interference RNA technology to inhibit cell cycle inhibitors is a feasible and possible treatment in the future.

Recently the group have turned their attention to feline osteoarthritis, a very common disease in older cats, but which surprisingly has been overlooked in the field and is still widely believed not to be of clinical importance. They showed for the first time that osteoarthritis in cats, just as in other species, is a painful condition with serious welfare implications if not recognised and treated.

Indeed it is likely that feline osteoarthritis will be a much better model of human osteoarthritis than either the dog or the horse.

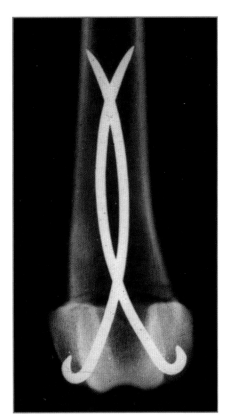

Rush-pinning of distal femoral fracture

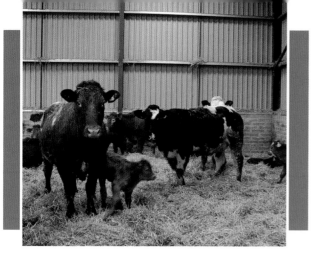

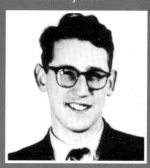
Animal health and production

Cattle diseases

Much of the farm animal research was developed from field investigations of diseases first identified in clinical cases referred to the School by many gifted practitioners, including George Barr, Ian MacMillan, Jim Begg, Brian Martin and Bill Jarrett's older brother Tom. These cases passed through the 'byres system' and were clinically evaluated and necropsied; then the farms from which they came were visited and disease pathogenesis was explored. It was a time when the link between clinicians and pathologists and their interdisciplinary approach to research led to a number of breakthroughs in understanding diseases of large as well as small animals.

Bovine respiratory diseases

The success of Dictol stimulated a particular interest in the plethora of ill-defined and poorly understood cases of bovine respiratory syndromes that were encountered during the development of the vaccine. Fog fever was a recurring enigmatic problem in the early 1960s and stimulated one of the most exciting and rewarding research programmes in bovine medicine led by Hugh Pirie and Ian Selman, working with PhD students Roger Breeze and Alisdair Wiseman and funded by the ARC.

Their clinico-pathological and epidemiological investigation on the nature and aetiology confirmed a condition of adult beef cattle, commonly confused with several others, causing acute respiratory distress and often death, that occurred when housed animals were transferred to lush grass pasture in autumn. The specific lesions in the lungs of fog fever cases were characterized by an acute respiratory syndrome due to pulmonary oedema, emphysema, hyaline membranes and alveolar epithelialisation due to proliferation of type II pneumonocytes. The prevailing view was that the condition was an allergy, perhaps to lungworm or *Mycopolyspora faeni*, the fungus which grows on mouldy hay.

It is now known to be due to intoxication by an excess of 3-methyl indole that resulted from fermentation in the rumen of the high concentration of tryptophan in the grass. Consequently, improved management systems were promoted to prevent the condition.

The group, strengthened by the mycologist Christine Dawson, began a detailed research programme throughout the 1970s to resolve issues about the pathogenesis of fog fever and the nature of the conditions with which it was confused.

Thus, fog fever was found not to be an allergy to lungworms, as had been suggested by others, although reinfection of cattle with lungworms was itself shown to be a significant economic problem with a distinct pathology characterised by multiple lymphoid nodules encapsulating dead larvae. Fog fever was also quite distinct from farmer's lung, a dangerous condition for both cattle and farm workers, which also underwent a major investigation by the respiratory team. Farmer's lung in cattle presents as a chronic wasting syndrome with a persistent cough in animals kept indoors and exposed to over-heated mouldy hay. It is a type III lung hypersensitivity allergy to the spores of thermophilic actinomycetes that are ideally sized to penetrate into the lung alveoli and that are released in huge numbers from the hay causing bronchiolitis obliterans.

The extensive contacts in the field that were established in these investigations in Scotland and northern England were fundamental in identifying new conditions in cattle. For example, a dramatic, severe form of infectious bovine tracheitis was discovered in cattle in Aberdeenshire from which the very virulent Strichen strain of bovine herpesvirus type I was isolated. This strain became a prototype virus that was subsequently used in research worldwide.

1995

The Weipers Centre for Equine Welfare opens.

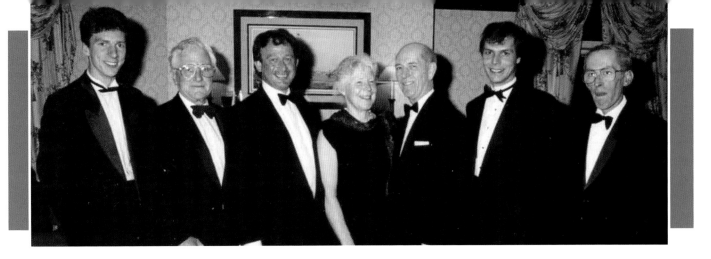

David Murphy, Gordon Hemingway, Jim Parkins, Mary Stewart, Norman Ritchie, Ewan Cameron and Graham Fishwick 1990

The severity of infection with this virus, and the spread of the disease to many other farms, was such that a modified live virus vaccine for IBR was permitted to be introduced into the UK for the first time for its control. Another example of being able to examine serious naturally-occurring diseases in depth was the transmission in calves of malignant catarrhal fever from a field case and a detailed study of its pathogenesis was undertaken by Ian Selman, Alisdair Wiseman, Norman Wright and Max Murray.

Further investigations of bovine respiratory disease revealed that 'calf pneumonia' did not have a single aetiology, like enzootic pneumonia in pigs, for example. Into the 1990s, Edna Allen, Robin Dalgleish, Alison Gibbs and Neil Watt joined the group and helped define other agents that were involved in natural infections. These were found to include parainfluenza type-3 virus, bovine respiratory syncytial virus, *Mycoplasma bovis* and *Pasteurella haemolytica*.

This large body of work over a period of thirty years had a major impact on improving the welfare of cattle in the UK. In addition, it provided a cohort of teachers with enormous experience of the natural occurrence of cattle diseases who influenced a generation of graduates of the School. This strong influence continues in the Scottish Centre for Production Animal Health and Food Safety at Garscube.

Neonatal mortality in calves

Neonatal diarrhoea caused heavy economic loss on dairy farms in the UK in the 1950s and 1960s. Bacteria were implicated but antibiotic therapy was often applied too late and was ineffective. Ted Fisher and colleagues developed enlightened rehydration therapy with electrolytes that provided effective treatment. In addition, in the 1960s and 70s, Ted with Douglas McEwan, Ian Selman and Clive Gay explored in detail the factors involved in neonatal death in calves.

They emphasised the crucial importance of colostrum intake by calves very soon after birth to provide adequate immunoglobulin levels to protect them from pathogenic bacteria. To aid treatment, they devised a simple method to determine the immunoglobulin concentration in the serum by a zinc sulphate turbidity test. Then, on farms throughout Scotland, they proposed management systems of feeding colostrum in order to provide consistent levels of absorbed immunoglobulin.

Ruminant nutrition

Gordon Hemingway joined the University Chemistry Department in 1953 and in 1960 moved to the Department of Animal Husbandry at the Veterinary School. He, along with Norman Ritchie and Jim Parkins, made major advances in ruminant nutrition from their base at Cochno University Farm and Research Centre.

They developed the first successful slow-release intra-ruminal boluses for cattle to prevent mineral deficiencies. These boluses were designed to lie in the reticulum of cattle and sheep whence they supplied vital dietary elements or drugs to the ruminant animal without the need for daily supplementation in feeds, which is often difficult for grazing stock.

The first unique sustained-release magnesium alloy ruminal bolus was patented by the University of Glasgow in 1966 and contains an alloy of magnesium, copper and aluminium which dissolves uniformly with time. It was licensed to aid the prevention of hypomagnesaemia in cows and ewes when grazing spring grass and also in the prevention of hypocalcaemia at calving time. Patent protection meant that the Glasgow device was the only such bolus on the world market for twenty years and it continues to have a large international market. The technology for the magnesium/aluminium/copper alloy, which was pivotal in the magnesium bolus, was also latterly (and still is) utilised by others in 'pulse release' anthelmintic drugs.

A further patented sustained release device invention, All-Trace boluses, also lies in the rumen-reticulum and is the only bolus that supplies a sustained dietary supplement of all seven trace elements and the three fat soluble vitamins required by ruminant animals. Many millions of these products have been sold worldwide, and specialised development of the trace element bolus continues.

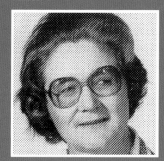

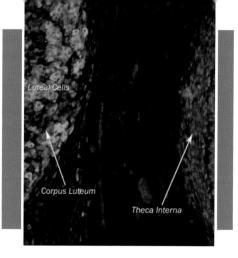

Fluoroscopy of ovarian follicles

Reproductive physiology

Over the past twenty years Peter O'Shaughnessy, Neil, Evans, Jane Robinson, Mike Harvey, Monika Mihm, Lindsay Robertson, Fiona Dowell and Ian Jeffcoate have studied the factors and mechanisms that control reproductive development and function. This is an area of particular importance as infertility still causes significant losses to both dairy and beef industries, and affects many human couples. In addition, it is now becoming clear many adult disorders have their origin in foetal life and that disruption of normal development, including reproductive development, will have significant knock-on effects for the quality of later life.

The programme of work has encompassed studies addressing testicular development which have largely used mouse models to identify how hormones secreted from the pituitary gland act to control growth of the testes.

To investigate the role of these hormones in development they used mice, generated by a colleague in Oxford, which either lack the hormones or lack the receptors for the hormones. From study of these mice they were able to show that one pituitary hormone acts to stimulate the early stages of spermatogenesis while another enables completion of germ cell production through increased androgen production.

These mouse models of infertility remain particularly potent tools for the study of reproduction and are being used to identify the mechanisms of hormone action in the testis. Models to address ovarian development and, specifically, how ovarian follicles grow and function before and after ovulation have been developed in the cow. These events are of particular agricultural relevance as they are affected by metabolic and other systemic and environmental influences. This means they are often severely compromised by the demands of lactation and management practices in the modern high-yielding dairy cow, leading to problems with fertility, and consequently dairy cow economics. The results of this work have identified new genes considered to be essential for healthy follicle development, and ovarian targets for the effects of severe energy deficit on both human and bovine ovarian follicle development. In addition to studies at the level of the gonads, this group have been interested in the means by which the steroids secreted from the ovary and the testis feedback on the central nervous system to control reproductive function. Their work in this area, which has primarily used sheep as a model species, has contributed to our knowledge of the roles of the neurotransmitters pro-opiomelanocortin, met-enkephalin, galanin, dopamine and neuropeptide Y on the reproductive axis. The group has also built up a significant reputation with regard to the effects of the environment experienced during development and its potential role in adult disease.

This work has again used mouse and ovine animal models, and through collaboration with colleagues in Aberdeen has also extended into studies in humans. In an ovine model animals are exposed to androgens during foetal development. This model results in masculinisation of female offspring which show some physiological features similar to those of polycystic ovarian syndrome in humans. Work on the effect of excessive androgen exposure during development parallels on-going research on the effects of developmental exposure to chemicals in our environment that can affect physiological systems. This work has shown that specific chemicals such as octylphenol, Bisphenol A, PCB 153 and PCB 118, all found within the environment, can affect the development and function of the hypothalamus, pituitary gland and uterus. Importantly, in collaboration with colleagues at the Universities of Aberdeen, Edinburgh and the James Hutton Institute, the group have also shown that many reproductive systems are significantly affected when they are exposed during foetal life to very low level mixtures of environmental toxicants.

To further understand the effect of environmental chemicals on reproduction they are also currently examining the effects that maternal lifestyle (and in particular the effects of maternal smoking) may have on the development of the foetal reproductive system.

1995

The James Herriot Library officially opened by Jim Wight, the author's son.

79

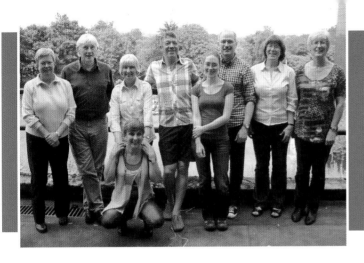

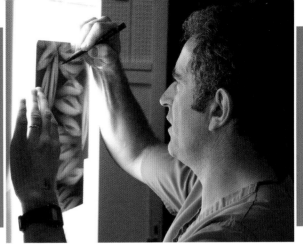

Physiology group 2012

Martin Sullivan examines salmon spine X-ray

Maternal smoking remains a major health problem: in Scotland: over twentyfive percent of women smoke during pregnancy and this figure rises to over sixty percent in the most deprived social categories. An additional aspect is that a number of the chemicals such as dioxin and cadmium in cigarette smoke are also potential environmental pollutants. So understanding how maternal smoking affects foetal development provides clues to how environmental pollutants may be acting during pregnancy. Their data so far have shown that maternal smoking specifically inhibits expression of a specific protein in the developing testis. It is known that this protein is required for normal testicular development and this may be a mechanism by which maternal smoking affects post-natal fertility in males. This later body of work has clearly shown that events experienced during prenatal development can affect the reproductive system and, potentially, other physiological systems such as those that regulate metabolism in later life.

The group is also leading research into the effects of alterations in reproductive hormone levels at later life stages. This work has resulted in the identification of changes in smooth muscle function that might contribute to the development of incontinence in females after they have been subjected to large changes in reproductive hormones.

This might occur, for example, in post-menopausal women or in bitches after they have been spayed.

Aquaculture

Aquaculture is the fastest growing of all the food-producing industries: in 2010 more than half of the fish and shellfish consumed in the world were derived from cultured species. By 2011, in Scotland salmon farming was of greater export value than beef, sheep and dairy combined and second only to whisky. Clearly this is a livestock production area where the veterinary profession plays a vital role. Much of this growth throughout the world is based on pioneering work begun at the Glasgow Veterinary School in the 1960s. Since then, Glasgow graduates have made significant contributions to that success in many countries.

In 1967, Glasgow was the first UK veterinary school to develop the subject of fish pathology. Much of the basic work on our understanding of the inflammatory and infectious processes in fish emanated from the Pathology Department. The principal scientist involved was Ron Roberts who, collaborating with others, made the School the UK centre for such work.

Inspired by this success, the Nuffield Foundation decided to establish a UK centre for the subject. Given the already overcrowded facilities in Glasgow it was decided to locate this on the new campus of the University of Stirling with Ron Roberts as Director and Sir William Weipers as the Chairman of its Management Board, with the intention of maintaining close links between the two centres.

The Institute of Aquaculture was established in Stirling in 1972 and grew to be the largest in the world. The strong collaborative links between the Glasgow School and the Stirling Institute have continued. Thus, in 1980 Ron Roberts led an international mission to investigate an economically damaging pandemic of rice field fishes in South-East Asia which was found to be caused by a new highly pathogenic Aphanomyces species. In this study, working with David Onions, they discovered the first retrovirus of fish, which promoted the pathogenicity of the fungal infection.

More recently, projects have involved Mike Stear and the parasitology group; and Martin Sullivan, using X-ray imaging has played a major part in a series of investigations of spinal deformities in fast-growing salmon with the result that this important condition affecting fish welfare has largely been eliminated in both Europe and Chile.

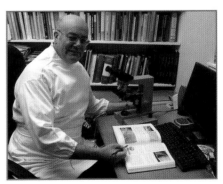

Ron Roberts

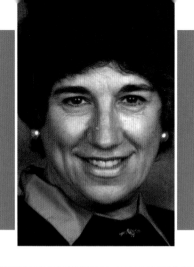

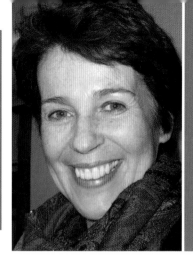

Maureen Bain

Maureen's research interests focus mainly on avian reproduction and specifically on egg formation and structure, and the functional properties of the oviduct in various domesticated species, with particular emphasis on the shell forming region.

Over the past twenty years she has developed an interdisciplinary line of research looking at novel methods for assessing egg and eggshell quality through international collaborations with such diverse groups as engineers and molecular biologists.

Sally Solomon   Maureen Bain

Poultry research

When the British Egg Marketing Board suggested that the public should 'Go to work on an egg' the poultry unit at the Glasgow School did literally that! In 1972 Sally Solomon, who was a postgraduate student of Bob Aitken, began a long career in the broad area of egg quality in birds and reptiles out of which the Poultry Unit developed.

It was because of its unique approach to egg quality in commercial birds (ducks, breeder and layer chickens, quail, and turkeys) that the Unit received international recognition. The group first described and categorised the range of structural variants found within the shells of today's modern hybrids and how these were affected by a wide range of management factors.

The range of technologies applied was extensive and included, in addition to its fundamental tools of light microscopy and scanning and transmission electron microscopy, the new techniques of confocal and laser-scanning microscopy. To encourage cooperation between industry and academia, the unit developed the Egg Quality Workshop series. These two-day courses were attended by poultry farmers, geneticists and management, and by displaying the abilities of the Unit and its application to industrial concerns many research contracts were established.

The focus on shell quality was extended to reptiles by a joint venture between Sally and the Cayman Island Turtle Farm, funded by the Royal Society. Thereafter the research field widened to include investigations on the breeding success of wild turtles in Padre Island, Florida and in Cyprus (both Greek and Turkish). The latter studies led to the formation of the Glasgow University Turtle Conservation Expedition, an inter-university summer research programme for undergraduates. The project continues from the University of Exeter under the direction of Brendan Godley and Annette Brodick, both of whom received their doctorates from Glasgow Veterinary School in this field of study.

But the unit spread its influence beyond science: in 1999 Sally Solomon curated her first exhibition of art inspired by electron microscopy, in the Hunterian Museum.

Sally was appointed to Professor of Poultry Science in 1995, the first female Professor in the Vet School as part of the University.

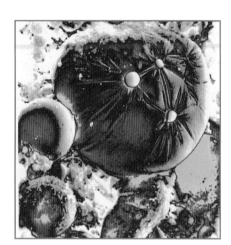

Electron microscopy of eggshell

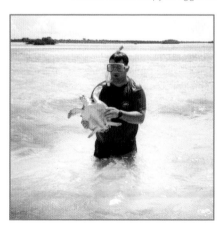

Brendan Godley BVMS 1994

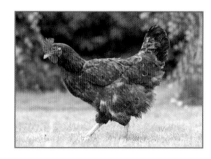

1999
Andrea Nolan becomes Dean, the first female Dean of a UK veterinary school.

81

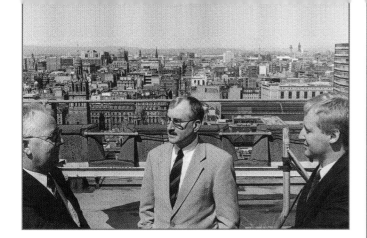

Max Murray, George Gettinby and Stuart Reid, Strathclyde University 1997

Veterinary Informatics and Epidemiology

In the 1970s descriptive epidemiology was becoming an important recognised addition to the understanding and control of veterinary diseases worldwide, and was commonly used to manage the life cycle of parasites of veterinary species. The subject had started to attract the attention of a growing number of veterinary schools across Europe and Northern America.

It was Glasgow Veterinary School that was to pioneer modern veterinary epidemiology for research in the UK veterinary schools with its focus on statistical, computer and mathematical modelling methods for the better understanding of parasitic populations. The early work of Jimmy Armour in the 1970s and 80s and the study of nematode populations in sheep and cattle populations required the analysis of worm counts in different life stages to assess the impact of the increasing number of new anthelmintic treatments available at this time.

By the beginning of the 1980s Jimmy Armour had brought together key UK players in the quantitative domain including George Gettinby, a young statistician at the University of Strathclyde, and Max Murray who in 1985 laid the foundations between the two Universities for a joint initiative in Veterinary Informatics and Epidemiology (VIE).

The inclusion of computer and information scientists brought the added dimension of informatics and the potential to deliver models, decision support and expert systems based on clinical data. Computer science contributions were provided by Crawford Revie an epidemiological information scientist from the University of Strathclyde. A proof of concept business plan established EqWISE as the universities first e-commerce site. Building on this early equine focus, ten productive years of collaboration with various international organisations including the University of Sydney added to the international reach of the new research group.

Richard Dixon BVMS 1993

While an impecunious PhD student in the Small Animal Medicine Department, Richard Dixon spotted an opportunity to supplement his grant and set up a small out-of-hours veterinary service for local practices. This proved so successful that he realised there was a great opportunity in a wider market. The public and profession were both changing and he had spotted a gap in the market. On the one hand, pet owners were looking for increasingly good care for their pets irrespective of the time of day or night. Secondly, the make-up of the profession was rapidly evolving: vets were expecting a better work life balance, out-of-hours work was becoming less popular, and the profession was increasingly staffed by women, many of whom wished to work part-time. Thus he founded 'Vets Now Ltd', a dedicated out-of-hours emergency and critical care service. But with no premises or staff, no business training or funding, there was much work to do.

Richard sold his long-term student flat in White Street to raise the initial capital. He then negotiated with the PDSA in Shamrock Street to use their premises in return for a rental and caring for their clients out-of-hours. The business was launched in December 2001. And it flourished: within eighteen months Vets Now had opened clinics in Bristol, Gateshead and Swansea. By 2012 the company had amassed more than fifty sites across the length and breadth of the UK. Caring for more than 100,000 patients every year with a turnover approaching £30M, and covering for approximately 1500 daytime veterinary surgeons, Vets Now has become one of the largest employers of veterinary surgeons and veterinary nurses in the UK. In 2006 Richard won the Young Alumnus of the Year award.

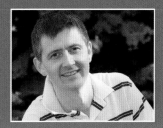

The collaboration between the Universities of Glasgow and Strathclyde was recognised by the appointment of Stuart Reid to the joint chair of Veterinary Informatics and Epidemiology in 1997 and the signing of a Synergy memorandum of agreement between the respective principals, Sir Graeme Davies and Sir John Arbuthnott in 1998. New epidemiological areas flourished with contributions and collaborations with Sandy Love, Chris Little, Tom Irwin, Ian McKendrick, Giles Innocent and more recently Louise Kelly. Over the next decade Stuart Reid led the VIE group in new directions. In the late 1990s a strategic liaison with Mark Woolhouse at the University of Edinburgh and George Gunn of the Scottish Agricultural College (SAC) was established bringing the veterinary and statistical skills of the Glasgow and SAC scientists together with the mathematical approach of the Edinburgh group (Louise Mathews). The group now focused on *E. coli* O157 and other zoonotic pathogens. In 2006 and with the passing of the local veterinary leadership to Dominic Mellor and notably the arrival of Dan Haydon, there was further evolution and a new identity. Combining the strengths of epidemiology with the ecological thinking of the life scientists the scope of work was considered much more appropriately as Population and Ecosystem Health and the multi-Faculty initiative was encapsulated in the Boyd Orr Centre.

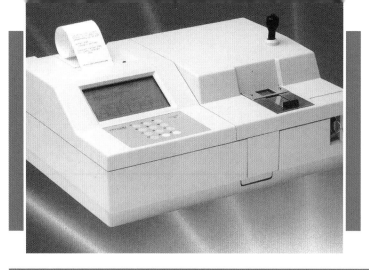

Vet Test 8008

Diagnostics

Point of care analysers

Roger Clampett, an innovative clinical biochemist and engineer with a compelling interest in point-of-care diagnostics, conceived a fully automated analyser that could be used in veterinary practice laboratories. He based himself in the Medicine Department in 1987 and worked on its commercial development with a multidisciplinary team which included Max Murray, Chris Little, Brian Wright, Ronnie Barron, the head of the biochemistry and haematology laboratories in the School, George Gettinby, technologist June Downs and software developer Steve Hazlewood.

It was a completely new concept in point-of-care blood chemistry analysers and included a unique software package 'The Biochemical Thermometer' employing the Glasgow Clinical Biochemical Database. It was found that the use of 'percentiles' to indicate by how much the result was abnormal, provided a much more informative picture of the clinical condition of the patient than existing methods. The result was the VT8008 analyser.

The VT8008 proved to be a huge commercial success and in 1991 was sold to the US veterinary supply company, IDEXX. By mid-2011 there were 50,000 of these analysers in the field which had tested samples from fifty million patients.

The VS 2000/ the HemaTek 2001 Blood Analysis System for animals, and the ESR Plus and Bilirubin Plus for Humans, were then launched in 2000. This instrumentation received the prestigious SMART Award (Small Funding Merit Award for Research and Technology) in 1992.

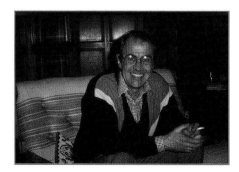

Roger Clampett

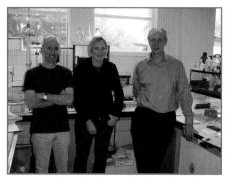

Chris McComb, Caroline Hogarth and David Eckersall

Acute phase proteins

A major research area in the School over the recent decades has been in the development, validation and application of assays for acute phase proteins (APP) by David Eckersall in collaboration with colleagues in the School including the companion and production animal clinics and Veterinary Diagnostic Services, and abroad. His laboratory has pioneered the use of specific protein assays in diagnostic biochemistry for veterinary medicine and methods to measure the APP. These assays were originally developed for research purposes and are now being transferred to commercial production for use in diagnostic laboratories worldwide and should be available for use in every veterinary clinic in the near future.

Among the significant advances that have been made by the laboratory is the development of a novel biochemical test for the measurement of haptoglobin in all species. Haptoglobin is the major marker of innate immunity in serum for cattle and sheep and the assay is in use on a global basis to identify the presence of clinical and subclinical infectious disease in these species.

1999
The 50th anniversary of amalgamation with the University of Glasgow.

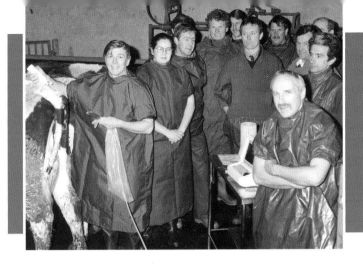

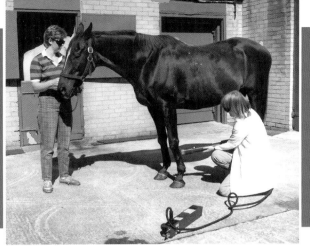

Another finding was that APP are synthesized in cows with mastitis. Work is continuing to establish whether measuring the concentration of these biomarkers of disease will have advantages in the diagnosis of this economically important disease of dairy cows.

Significant advances are also being made in the application of the APP in the diagnosis of disease in companion animals. Susan Duthie, working with virologist Diane Addie, discovered that measuring the serum concentration of alpha-1 acid glycoprotein (AGP) is valuable in the diagnosis of FIP. While a raised level is not specific for FIP, it helps distinguish this disease from other clinically similar conditions, so that the AGP assay has become an integral part of the algorithm for laboratory diagnosis.

The alteration in serum concentration of canine APPs have also been investigated in a variety of infectious, inflammatory and neoplastic diseases by various clinicians including Jo Morris and Rory Bell and have been valuable in the detection of the innate immune and inflammatory reactions, and subsequent monitoring of responses to treatment.

The research produced by the laboratory has led to the formation of a university spinout company, ReactivLab Ltd which was acquired by the Avacta Group in 2010. It focuses on the commercialisation of APP assays, with the aim of developing systems so they can be transferred to diagnostic laboratories around the world.

Ultrasonography

In 1958 Ian Donald, the Professor of Midwifery and Gynaecology at the University of Glasgow, first used ultrasound in obstetrical and gynaecological clinical diagnosis. Working with engineer Tom Brown and a young registrar John MacVicar in the newly-built Queen Mother's Maternity Hospital, they launched the use of this technology in human diagnostic medicine. As a result, a number of companies set up in Livingston to develop production models of diagnostic ultrasound equipment. In the mid-1980s, Jack Boyd, the Professor of Clinical Veterinary Anatomy, with the gift of an off line scanner from medical colleagues began developing this non-invasive technology for veterinary use. (Although Jack Boyd may be best remembered by graduates for his ability to drink a pint of beer whilst standing on his head!)

The possibility of new markets influenced the manufacturers in Livingston so that new equipment became available at Garscube, which was of mutual benefit in progressing modification of equipment for routine veterinary use. Charities such as the Home of Rest for Horses, who were eager to advance diagnostic research by non-invasive techniques, were attracted to support the ultrasound unit. From modest beginnings with borrowed equipment the ultrasound unit at the School became a centre for ground breaking work in the use of diagnostic ultrasound in animals.

Dealing with tendon tearing and rupture in high performance horses coupled with the controversy surrounding the use of firing or blistering which had plagued the veterinary profession for decades, the ability to detect and categorise tendon lesions in horses using ultrasonography provided the perfect solution to investigate and problem solve. Celia Marr, 1985 graduate, was one of the early leaders in the UK in this field. She then extended the use of ultrasound into cardiac and abdominal diagnosis in both large and small animals to provide a diagnostic service to the clinicians in the Hospital.

Probably the major area for advancement was in reproductive studies so that the School became a leading centre for reproductive research as well as offering professional development training to a large section of the practicing veterinary profession in reproductive diagnostic work. Added to this were training sessions for practitioners throughout the UK and overseas in the use of the many applications of ultrasound in both small and large animals including fish and reptiles. Staff members included Jack Boyd, Alison King and Calum Paterson, the latter recently retiring in 2011 after fortyone years of service in the University! By having the technology available to undergraduates in the early stages of the course a new generation of veterinary graduates was being produced who were fully conversant with the multitude of applications of non-invasive diagnostic ultrasound.

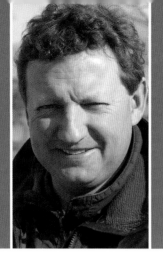

Mark Johnston BVMS 1983

Mark, former Young Alumnus of the year in 2001, was recognised for his outstanding contribution to the horse racing world both as a trainer and a vet. He was named Flat Trainer of the year in 1994, and in 1997 he broke the record for the fastest 1000 Flat victories by a trainer in Britain.

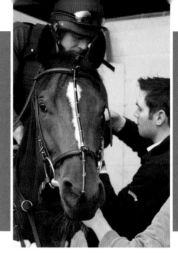

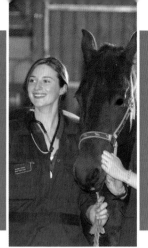

Dynamic respiratory endoscopy in the horse

The introduction of dynamic respiratory endoscopy is one of the most exciting innovations in equine medicine in recent years. In collaboration with the pioneering French endoscopy company Optomed, Patrick Pollock and clinicians were the first to use and validate this equipment in horses that were presented for investigation of poor performance or abnormal respiratory noise. The equipment, at the time the only marketable version of its kind in the world, allows the acquisition of images of the equine pharynx and larynx under normal exercise conditions and thus immediately eliminated the need for high-speed treadmill endoscopy.

There are many conditions that affect the upper respiratory tract of horses, some of which are known to be dynamic in nature: that is, that they are either more severe or occur only during exercise, such as idiopathic laryngeal hemiplegia and intermittent dorsal displacement of the soft palate. The endoscope is inserted in one nostril and held in place on a specially designed bridle while a pack containing a wireless transmitting device is attached to a saddle-cloth, and the examining vet has a hand-held video display and control box. The fact that it is possible to examine the pharynx and larynx during exercise conditions allows veterinary students to visualise dynamic airway disease as it happens, monitoring the airway live in the training environment; one student remarked that it was 'almost like being in the pharynx'!

Collaboration with the Moredun Research Institute

Since the relocation of the Moredun Research Institute from the Veterinary College in Glasgow to Edinburgh in 1922, the two institutions have collaborated closely on a large number of research projects and many Glasgow veterinary students have gained research experience through vacation scholarships at the Institute. This relationship was formalised in May 2006 when a Memorandum of Understanding was signed by the Principal of the University of Glasgow and the Director of the Moredun Institute.[137]

Current projects include research on jaagsiekte sheep retrovirus which causes ovine pulmonary adenocarcinoma, a contagious lung cancer in sheep. Supervised by David Griffiths (Moredun) and Massimo Palmarini (Glasgow University) and funded by a Scottish Funding Council Strategic Research Development Grant to the Moredun, Glasgow University and the Roslin Institute, this project is investigating the virus-host interactions of JSRV and infected cells by identifying the role of cellular proteins in controlling virus replication. The knowledge gained in cell culture will be applied *in vivo* to the control of JSRV in sheep.[138]

Since 1976 the post of Scientific Director of Moredun Research Institute has been held successively by Glasgow graduates; Bill Martin, 1976-85; Ian Aitken, 1985-97; Quintin McKellar, 1997-2004 and Julie Fitzpatrick, 2004-present. Julie's secondment to the post of Professor of Food Security within the College of Medical, Veterinary and Life Sciences at the University in 2011 has further strengthened the close ties between the Glasgow Vet School and the Moredun Research Institute.

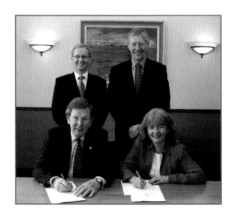

Stuart Reid, John Jeffrey, Muir Russell and Julie Fitzpatrick

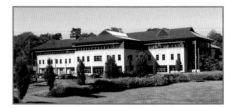

Moredun Research Institute

| 1999

The Faculty is accredited by the American Veterinary Medical Association.

85

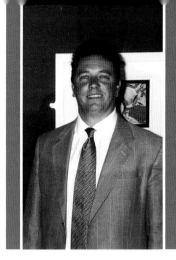

Douglas Hutchison BVMS 1980

Douglas Hutchison worked in large animal practice for three years before becoming technical advisor for a pharmaceutical company, moved into sales and marketing and finally becoming general manager. After two years with a venture capital group he and his wife Pippa set up Veterinary Business Development which grew to be one of the most successful media and publishing companies in the sector. Douglas has served as a member of the RCVS Communications board, as a trustee of the Veterinary Surgeons' Health Support Programme, and a director of VetAid. He is chairman of a number of companies and most recently was co-opted onto the Board of Trustees of the Royal Zoological Society of Scotland.

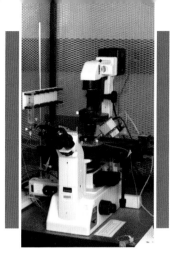

Equipment at CIDS

Veterinary Diagnostic Services

When the whole School was finally located at Garscube in 1969, the laboratory diagnostic services that supported clinical work, teaching and research were scattered among individual departments but gradually, in a series of steps, these subjects were brought together to form the present Veterinary Diagnostic Services. The main impetus for this process was to improve efficiency by bringing together all of the available technical expertise. In addition, as there was a growing demand from veterinary practitioners and pharmaceutical companies for the expertise that was accruing as a result of the burgeoning basic and clinical research in the School, there were opportunities for commercialisation.

Indeed, the feline and canine virology laboratories as well as clinical biochemistry and haematology already had commercial arms which provided a useful income stream to support further research and development. An association, albeit short, with the Bloxham company in 1998 afforded an opportunity to co-locate haematology and clinical chemistry.

A further reorganisation of space in the preclinical building provided a modern refurbished laboratory for these subjects, and also incorporated histopathology.

Now all of the laboratory-based diagnostic facilities, including bacteriology, parasitology and virology, are integrated in Veterinary Diagnostic Services which offers a comprehensive range of aids to clinical diagnosis to the School and to veterinary practitioners throughout the UK and abroad. The Clinical Director is the Professor of Veterinary Pathology, Janet Patterson-Kane and the Academic Heads of Clinical Pathology and Infectious Diseases are Hayley Haining and Libby Graham respectively.

Commercialism and technology transfer

The School has had a strong tradition of commercialising the outputs of its research stretching back to the 1950s and the launch of the Dictol vaccine. That tradition has been maintained over the following decades with many commercial successes which have provided crucial support for the School's development.

In the late 1990s the School's role in commercialisation was further enhanced when as part of the Equine Hospital development, commercial incubator space was included as an integral part of the new building. Managed by Sylvia Morrison a large number of university spin-out companies have been provided with essential space in which to develop into independent entities. This venture was the first of its type in the University. In 2001 the Vet School also played a leading role in establishing the Centre for Integrated Diagnostic Systems (CIDS) Biomedical Incubator based at Gilmorehill. Both facilities were supported by the University, Scottish Enterprise and the ERDF. Both Units were highly successful. By 2012, twentyfive of the twentynine businesses that have been spun out by the University had used the foregoing incubator facilities, with the waiting list closed for non-Glasgow University companies. Collectively, the companies spun out of the University with infrastructure support from the Vet School have created well in excess of 500 high-tech jobs in Scotland, adding significant value to the Scottish economy.

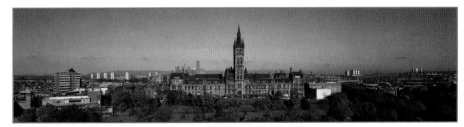

University of Glasgow

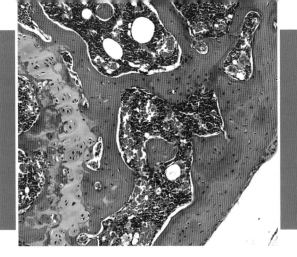

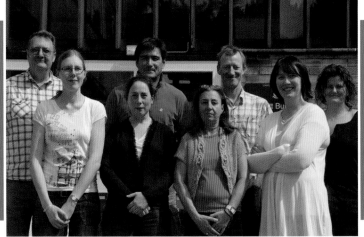

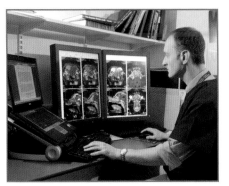

Gawain Hammond, assessing MRI scans

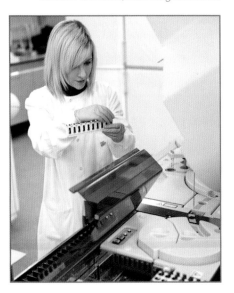

Conclusions

Glasgow Veterinary School justifiably prides itself on its research and has excelled in many spheres. In 1988, Glasgow was awarded the highest Research Assessment Exercise (RAE) of a UK veterinary school. The RAE is a bench-marking exercise to measure the quality of research conducted by universities across the UK and is an internationally recognised barometer of quality.

This position was retained in 1992 and 1996 and joint best was achieved in 2001 and 2008.[139] The School has also consistently had one of the highest levels of research income of any UK veterinary school and has made a major contribution to the recognition that, on the basis of citation analysis, Scotland leads the world in veterinary and animal science publications (in all other areas of biomedicine the world leader is the USA).

In the old College, there had been little opportunity for research. However, through the foresight of Sir William Weipers who had the vision to establish outstanding multidisciplinary teams of researchers working within the context of 'One Health, One Medicine' a powerful research tradition was established and flourished. The veterinary scientists that he recruited attracted bright young graduates, who in turn consolidated and expanded their achievements to the present day.

Thus the Glasgow *esprit de corps* developed by Weipers has been maintained and enhanced. Weipers' genius was not only to gather the best of men and women, but also to generate and sustain an environment of entrepreneurship and creativity based on interdisciplinary interactions. It is this framework that has continued and expanded to this day as reflected by the large teams of veterinary scientists in many disciplines. Innovations such as The Henry Wellcome Building for Comparative Medical Sciences in 2004 and the MRC Centre for Virus Research, the largest virology centre in the UK, to be opened in 2014, ensures that Glasgow Veterinary School's pre-eminence remains firmly embedded on the research and innovation map of the world.

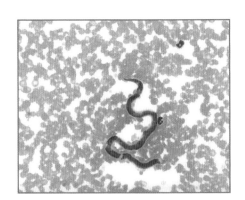

Heartworm

2001

The Weipers Centre for Equine Welfare surgical suites are completed.

87

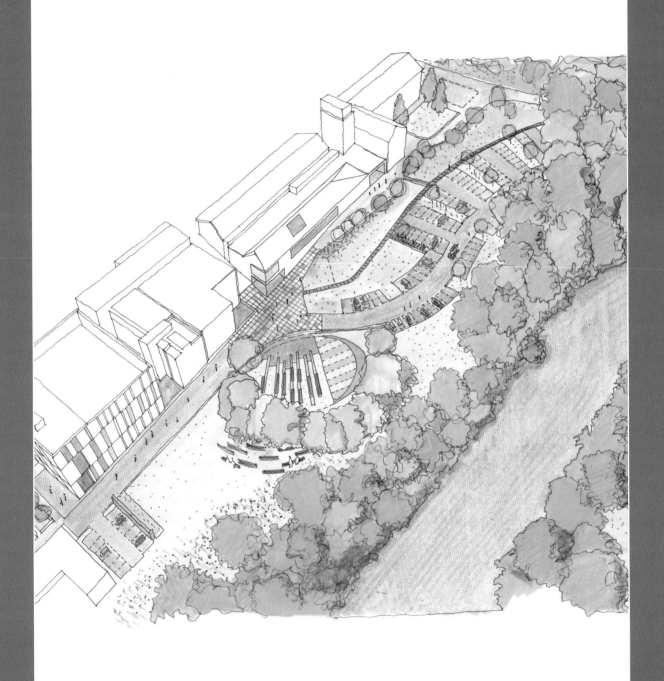

Vision for the future at Garscube, architects' impression 2012

Chapter Five

Bricks and Mortar

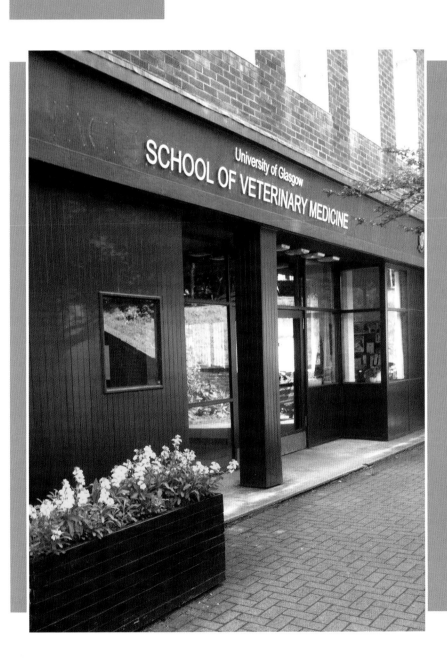

Pastures new: The Veterinary Hospital at Garscube

Weipers' vision could only be realised by building new facilities. Garscube Estate in Bearsden on the northwest edge of Glasgow had been obtained by the University under the guidance of the Principal, Sir Hector Hetherington in 1948 to expand the University as the Gilmorehill site was becoming overcrowded. This was to be the site for the future development of the Veterinary School.

Garscube House

In 1948, the University purchased Garscube House and the surrounding land from Sir George Campbell of Succoth (a property in Cardross) for £16,000. The property had belonged to the Campbell family since 1687 when it was acquired by John Campbell of Succoth from Sir John Colquhoune of Luss. It had originally been granted in 1250 to Umphredus de Kilpatrick by Maldwin, Earl of Lennox as part of the lordship of Colquhoune. The house at Garscube was initially used as a Glasgow residence by the Earls of Montrose. The Campbell family had close connections with the University. John Campbell's great grandson, Ilay Campbell, was a student in the early 1750s.

Ilay Campbell later became a very successful advocate and was Lord President of the Court of Session from 1789 to 1808. He became Rector of the University from 1799 to 1801 and was created a Baronet on his retirement which he spent at Garscube. He died in 1823 at the age of 89. His son Sir Archibald pulled down the old house and commissioned the well-known country house architect William Burn to build a sumptuous new home. Completed in 1827, the house faced south overlooking landscaped gardens beside the River Kelvin which were laid out to take advantage of the steep escarpment on the west bank of the river. It had been the University's intention to keep Garscube House but in 1954 it was found to be riddled with dry rot and to the disappointment of William Weipers, it was decided that the building would be demolished.[140]

Sir James Black speaking at a 'Home of Rest for Horses' event 1995 'Bill Weipers was dynamic in every sense of the word. Literally, he lived life on the trot – impatient to meet life in full. From his terrier-like face (I never saw him give up on anything), his piercing blue eyes, shaded by bushy eyebrows, penetrated the world around him.

I worked with him for eight years and learned to love that man. I saw him plan and build the new School at Garscube. He had two abiding interests in life: sick animals and healthy trees. He brought both of them together at Garscube. Indeed, the architect's favourite site for the building was moved thirty yards to the east at Bill's insistence – to save a marvellous sequoia.'

Garscube is a beautiful 200 acre estate, which had belonged to the Campbell family, located on the city boundary and bisected by the River Kelvin on its way to the Clyde. It was perfect for the evolution of the one-site strategy for the Veterinary School. Another advantage of Garscube was that it was only three miles from the Gilmorehill campus, the Medical School and the Bioscience and Engineering Departments with which major collaboration would evolve over the years. The green fields of Garscube provided much needed space for expansion of the clinical departments and facilities for research.

Weipers worked closely with the architects Gillespie, Kidd and Coia in developing the Veterinary Hospital to provide advanced teaching and research space, as well as hospital facilities to cater for referrals of clinical cases, essential for the new course. He was also able to indulge his enthusiasm for arboriculture by planting trees around the estate.[141] Although work began in 1950, by 1952 staff had entry only to the animal accommodation with the prospect of possessing two rooms by the end of the year. Kennel wards, loose boxes and haylofts were used by staff and students for lectures and as a refectory.

The Veterinary Hospital building, now known as the McCall Building, was officially opened in 1954 by the Secretary of State for Scotland, the Rt Hon James Stuart, MVO MC (later Viscount Stuart of Findhorn).[142] The building housed the main administration block, offices, lecture rooms including a large assembly hall, laboratory space, radiography and operating theatres, library, dining and common rooms.[143]

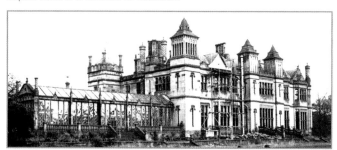

Garscube house

It was agreed that departments would move to the new site from Buccleuch Street in a phased programme over approximately ten years. The first new building to be constructed was the Veterinary Hospital, now a listed building, which was completed in 1954.

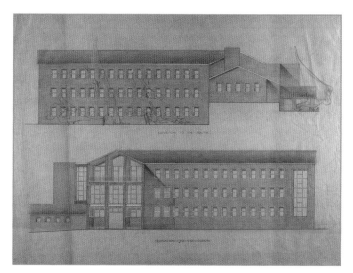

Plans of McCall building

Catriona Dunn (Cowan) reminisces on the early days at Garscube

'There's a pawn shop on a corner in Pittsburgh, Pennsylvania…' was being sung by the kennel maid on 5 May, 1952, as I started my first job at the age of 21 as Assistant Secretary to Mrs. Keith ('K-E-I- T-H' as she always spelled it out on the phone) at the University Veterinary Hospital in Garscube Estate. I hadn't wanted an officey-type job and Garscube, in its early days, exceeded my wildest dreams.

The office was a dog kennel; the professional staff, all four of them, Messrs. Sidney Jennings, Ian McIntyre, Donald Lawson, and Ian Lauder, shared a larger kennel which had a desk in each corner. About a year-and-a-half later, when I was Medicine and Surgery Departmental Secretary plus half of Pathology, the office was a desk in the Medicine/ Pathology laboratory in the hay loft.

Access was via a ladder from the PM Room underneath (which was itself a horse loose box), and through a hole in the ceiling. No health and safety at work in those days, thank goodness, for it was all GREAT FUN - and masses of work got done! Andy Waterson and Jimmy Murphy, the stockmen, would obligingly milk a cow to provide milk for our coffee. Nobody stood on ceremony under these circumstances and an atmosphere of friendly cooperation developed. If any friction did occur, the ever optimistic Camilla Colquhoun (now Guthrie) would say 'It'll all blow over'. She wasn't quite so sure when she overheard Dr Ian McIntyre say 'We are giving books this Christmas'! The building of the new Vet School took place around us and only final year students attended lectures at Garscube at that time. Firm friendships were made among the small numbers of staff, which endure to this day.

Mary Stewart was part of the shift to Garscube and was later a member of the small team that laid the foundations of the new School. She came to the stark contrast of Buccleuch Street in Glasgow in 1950 from the lovely campus of Cornell where she graduated. She was the house surgeon in a 'trio of dogsbodies' which was made up of the only secretary Catriona Cowan, stockman Jimmy Murphy and herself.

'Willy Weipers, though frantically busy as Dean, always had time for people, and was curious and interested in everybody and everything.

I remember him ensuring that I was 'getting the proper nutrition' and bringing me intellectually stimulating books when I was in hospital for an appendix operation. He had a passion for trees, and designed the new buildings so that there was minimum disruption. At weekends he would be out in his old clothes and beret, digging and planting new trees. There was one occasion when a young student couldn't get his car started, and seeing someone working on the grounds, went over and asked him to help push, which he willingly did. The student was mortified when the 'gardener' gave the Dean's welcoming address to the new students.' [144]

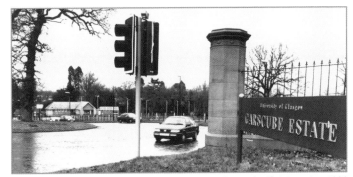

Garscube Estate gates 1998

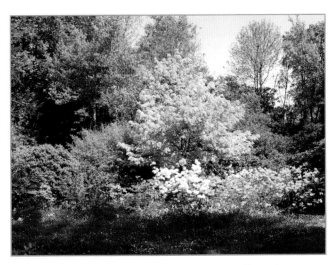

Garscube campus

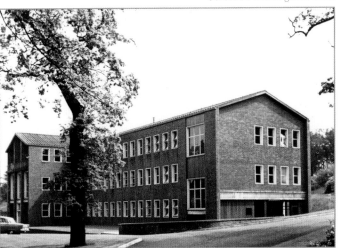

McCall building 1950s

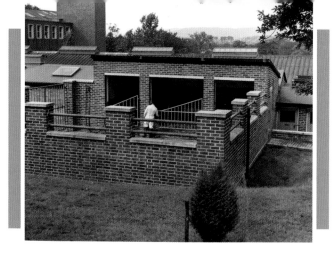

The Byres 1960s

Sir James Armour, reminisces.

'On returning to Glasgow Veterinary School in 1963 and comparing it to when I left in 1952 the most striking change was that veterinary education now took place in a research-motivated environment. Evidence based medicine was in place long before the term became the norm!

The level of collaboration between different disciplines was high and the emphasis was on multi-disciplinary teams.

At that time Glasgow was well ahead of other UK and European vet schools in its research ethos. There were many success stories and I was fortunate to be part of the group researching parasitic disease of livestock such as dictyocauliasis, ostertagiasis and fascioliasis. The fact that Glasgow vet science regularly topped the RAE ratings in the late 1980s through to 2001 reflected the quality of the work, the Vet School being based almost entirely on one site, at Garscube Estate, undoubtedly contributed to these successes and bolstered team spirit.' [145]

Clinical, pre and para - clinical facilities

The Byres

The food animal buildings, the 'byres' as they were affectionately known, were largely unaltered from the time the School was relocated to the Garscube Estate in the 1950s until radical developments in 2010. They consisted of three 'streets' of housing. On the bottom were seven or so loose boxes (one modified to a calf house). Up the stairs to the middle street there was a holding byre where cases were tied up for student and intern examination. Finally there was the top street which had a cattle yard and additional pens. At the side was the stockman's bothy, a sometimes bawdy place! Handling facilities were rudimentary but mirrored those on many farms.

But the 'byres' biggest boon was that they were close to the post mortem room. As a result of this liaison between clinicians, pathologists and other paraclinical departments it was here that the Faculty's reputation as one of the world's leading veterinary schools was forged.

The period starting in the 1950s and running through to the 1970s, when many major personalities held sway, was pivotal to the development of the modern school. Bill Jarrett, Bill Mulligan, Jimmy Armour, Sidney Jennings, Ian McIntyre, Ian Selman, Alasdair Wiseman, Peter Hignett, Ted Fisher, Donald Lawson and, of course, the then Dean Sir William Weipers were all larger than life. There are many more, but suffice to say it was a platform for many gifted teachers and veterinarians many of whom such as Roger Breeze and Lyall Petrie, went on to other parts of the world. 'Referred' cases passed through the 'byres system' and were clinically evaluated and necropsied, then farms were visited and disease pathogenesis explored. Despite the basic design and lack of development of the fabric of the facility for many years it was a golden period for interaction between clinicians and pathologists in both teaching and research.

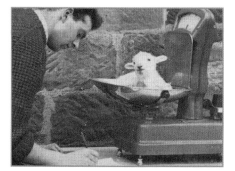

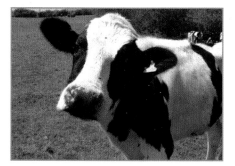

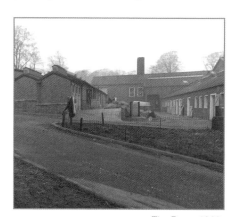

The Byres 1960s

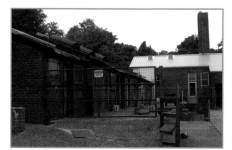

The Byres 2000s

2005

The Henry Wellcome Building for Comparative Medical Sciences opens at a cost of £7M.

93

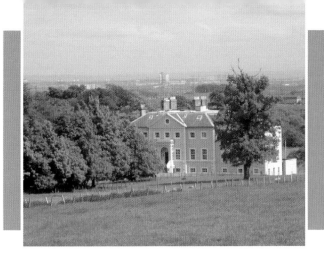

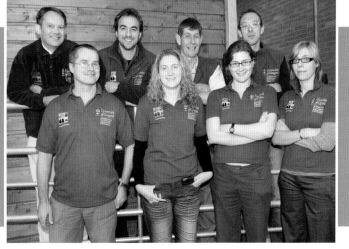

Cochno Estate

In 1954, the University of Glasgow purchased the 250 acre estate of Cochno, five miles to the northwest of the Veterinary Hospital. This provided farm facilities for teaching practical aspects of animal husbandry and veterinary preventive medicine. Plans were made to convert the house, a B-listed building, built around 1757 by John Adam, into a hostel for students but these never came to fruition. However, the estate provided the ideal environment for veterinary students to gain valuable hands-on experience.[146, 147] This followed a recommendation from the Loveday report to promote improvements in the training of students in farm animal husbandry and nutrition.

Extensive renovations to the house took place between 1992 and 2003, transforming it into a first class site for teaching and an excellent conference venue. The picturesque Cochno Estate is a site of special wildlife interest. The grounds include over 100 acres of woodlands and lochs with waterfalls and over three miles of inland water courses.[148] Scott Inglis was the first Professor of Animal Husbandry 1956 until his death in 1967.

He was responsible for the management of the Cochno facilities for many years until it was taken over by Gordon Hemingway, an animal scientist who joined the Department of Animal Husbandry in 1960 and was appointed to the Chair in 1969. Jim Parkins, an animal scientist, was Professor of Animal Health at the University and Director of The University Farm and Research Centre at Cochno from 1990 until his retirement in 2010. It was at Cochno that Gordon Hemingway, Norman Ritchie and Jim Parkins designed the first slow-release intra-ruminal boluses to prevent trace element mineral deficiencies in cattle.

Today, Cochno Farm extends to over 850 acres of grassland with five hundred breeding ewes, ninety dairy cows, a small beef herd and all the replacement and fat livestock. The Research Centre has expanded with new buildings able to accommodate a wide range of animals from quail to cattle. The farm has increased in size with new buildings to enhance the capacity for teaching and operational work.

Many great celebrations and events have taken place over the years at Cochno. It has featured in the film 'Regeneration' as a war hospital and provided a shed full of turkeys in the popular TV series, 'Taggart'![149] Sadly, in the spring of 2009, Cochno House was unexpectedly found to have extensive dry rot, wet rot and woodworm infestations and was closed for repairs.[150]

Netherton Farm

In the 1980s Netherton Farm became part of the School. It was owned by Glasgow City Council and had been used previously as a cattle holding facility. Situated on the banks of the Forth and Clyde Canal, it was within walking distance of the Veterinary School. The School used Dictol royalty funds to purchase the facility and it was useful for a number of years as additional cattle and sheep accommodation before the site was sold by the University for housing development.

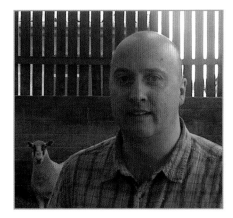

Peter Hastie, Director of Cochno Farm and Research Centre 2012

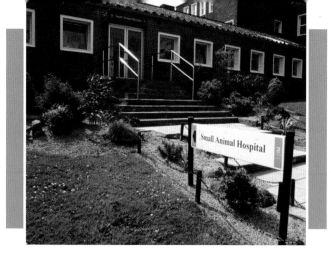

Small Animal Hospital 1980s-2009

The Small Animal Hospital

When the clinical departments moved to Garscube in 1952 the single-storey dog kennel block attached to the main building, along with the attached open–air dog runs behind, was a significant facility. The consultation rooms, two operating theatres, X-ray suite, pharmacy and other small animal clinical facilities were all on the ground floor of the main building. Clients had to use the main entrance door to the building. This arrangement remained in place for nearly thirty years until in the 1980s the increasing demand for referrals for companion animals required the small animal facilities to be refurbished and expanded. This involved the construction of a new two-storey building on the site of the open-air dog runs. On the ground floor new dog accommodation was built and on the second floor there was accommodation for student lockers and other facilities. (Later a third storey was added to house the Herriot Library). The old dog kennels were converted into a suite of consulting rooms and client waiting areas. These changes allowed the development of the lower floor of the main hospital building. In addition, an intensive care unit was established and ultrasound was relocated to the old large animal radiology suite.

The new small animal clinical facilities were officially opened in 1986 by John Parry, RCVS Junior Vice President. Several improvements were made to the hospital over the following decade such as refurbishment of the reception areas and installation of a dedicated clinical computed tomography (CT) scanner, the first in a UK veterinary school. Stuart Carmichael was appointed to the new post of Director of the Small Animal Hospital, and the Hospital was organised into a number of specialist units, making Glasgow unique in its wide range of referral services offered to vets in general practice.

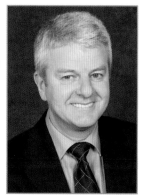

Stuart Carmichael

Robin Lee remembers,

'I moved from teaching Applied Anatomy at Liverpool to the Surgery Department at Glasgow in 1966. At that time Sir William Weipers was Professor and Head of Department and the other staff were Donald Lawson, Jimmy Campbell, Bob Cook, David Weaver, Ian Griffiths, Ian Glen, Bob Wyburn and Brian Holroyd. Surgery occupied the bottom corridor of the main building along with a lecture theatre, the pharmacy and some administrative offices. Medicine was on the first floor and Animal Husbandry on the top floor; the pre-clinical building was still under construction.

Reproduction was part of the Surgery department but operated largely independently under the leadership of Peter Hignett with Hugh Boyd, Jean Renton and latterly Mike Harvey.

The consulting rooms were immediately inside the main door and clients waited under the main staircase. The single-storey extension to the main building housed the small animal kennels with outside runs and further up was the farm animal and equine accommodation. The large animal operating theatre was adjacent to the X-ray room and small animal theatres. This meant that following surgery horses had to be towed by tractor on a low trailer up to a recovery box on the 'top street'. Shortly after my arrival the development opposite the main building was commissioned and included a two-story refectory,

an office block for the department of surgery and for some peculiar reason a large animal operating theatre and recovery room at one side and a block of equine loose boxes at the other - so horses had still to be moved between the two down a narrow concrete runway, albeit conscious!

This allowed redevelopment of the large animal theatre into a radiology suite for both large and small animals and expansion of the small animal operating theatres. It also freed space in the bottom corridor for more small animal consultation rooms.

Staff changes during this time included Bob Cook to the Animal Health Trust, replaced by Gordon Baker; Bob Wyburn to Massey University resulting in my involvement in radiology; Ian Glen left for a position in industry to be replaced by Nick Dodman, and Melvyn Pond joined Jimmy Campbell in developing orthopaedics.

Other recollections include delivering lectures in the 'hay loft' above the medicine byres on middle street and having to justify the release of the simplest of surgical supplies from the 'pharmacist' Mr Maxwell'.

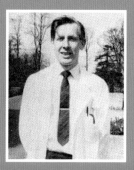

2006
Memorandum of understanding signed with the Moredun Research Institute.

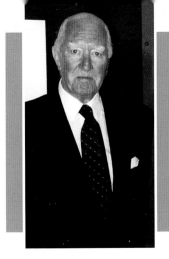
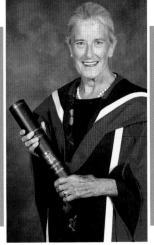

Forbes Macpherson   Alison Bruce, 2012

Planning for further major developments

Veterinary school development committee

A development committee, termed the 'A1 Project Committee', set up under the Deanship of Jimmy Armour and chaired by Max Murray had been established in 1989. In 1990 the University responded favourably to a 'Building and Information Communications Technology' proposal and funds were sought under the auspices of the University Development Office. In the first instance, this would be for the new equine facility and for a veterinary epidemiological informatics initiative. This advance resulted in a whole series of major new builds and developments over the next twenty years. Subsequently, this agreement was refined through the efforts of Dean Norman Wright so that in 2003 the A1 Project Committee became the University of Glasgow Veterinary Development Fund with the authority to prioritise projects, which then would be listed and supported by the full might of the Development and Alumni Office (DAO) of the University.[151] The DAO builds on relationships with alumni and friends worldwide and harnesses support for current and future projects. Increased student numbers and static Government funding had meant resources were being stretched. The threat of closure in 1988/89 and the huge response to the public campaign had demonstrated the overwhelming respect and affection for the Vet School at home and overseas. Forbes Macpherson, former Chancellor's Assessor was appointed Chairman of the Development Fund Advisory Board in 2003 and served in this capacity until December 2008. He explained that 'the Veterinary School Development Fund was committed to bridge the gap between state funding and the funding required to maintain the school's outstanding international reputation and continual improvements in building and equipment'.[152] The committee continues in this important work. The Veterinary School has the strongest history of fund-raising activity in the University to provide infrastructure, and most of the developments at the School have been achieved as a result of these efforts.

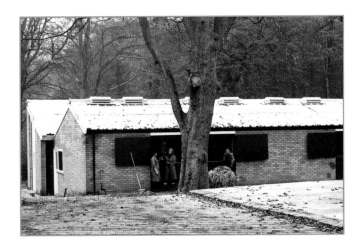

Old equine unit

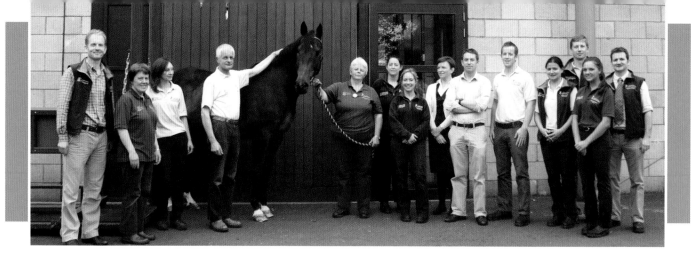

The Weipers Centre for Equine Welfare

Named after Sir William Weipers, construction on the first phase of the Weipers Centre for Equine Welfare was completed in 1995, costing £6M. Sandy Love, appointed Professor in 1995 and Head of the Division of Equine Studies, was one of the driving forces behind the ambitious project, a landmark achievement for the Vet School. In sharp contrast to the 'byres', there were absolutely no nostalgic feelings about the old equine 'facilities' such as they were. The medicine stables were down below the Henry Wellcome Building and had previously been pharmacology research stabling; the surgery stabling was next to the Stewart building; and the operating room was between the Stewart building and the refectory. X-ray and endoscopy facilities were shared with the old small animal hospital. Lameness examinations often took place in the staff car park where horses were loaded and unloaded. Further, there were no dedicated examination or treatment rooms: everything was just done in the stables. Essentially equine consultations, diagnostics and treatment areas were scattered and it was with great enthusiasm that fund-raising began in earnest for a new equine facility.

Equipped with the latest technology in diagnostic imaging, and incorporating a Sports Injury Clinic, the Centre was the first veterinary centre in Europe to make use of extended field of view ultrasonography for the improved diagnosis of musculoskeletal injuries.

In addition the facility had automated radiographic and fluoroscopic equipment and a gamma camera for improved nuclear scintigraphic diagnoses, all cutting edge equipment at that time. The diverse range of medical diagnostic tools included videoendoscopy, continuous ECG and echocardiography for the evaluation of cardiac abnormalities as well as laparoscopy to minimise invasive abdominal investigation. The Weipers Centre was officially opened by HRH Princess Royal in September 2001 following its final phase of construction. This phase included a surgical suite with twin operating theatres, one of which is dedicated to orthopaedic surgery, and an indoor lameness hall. There are two induction/recovery rooms with special padding, soundproofing and soft lighting. Images from the operating rooms can be relayed to the new lecture theatre for teaching purposes.

Funding for the project came from many sources including the Home of Rest for Horses (now known as The Horse Trust), the European Regional Development Fund, Merck & Co, the Hugh Fraser Foundation, Scottish Society for the Prevention of Cruelty to Animals, International League for the Protection of Horses (now known as World Horse Welfare), the Donkey Sanctuary, International Donkey Protection Trust and the Robertson Trust. Individuals, alumni, local groups, trusts, charities and businesses gave under the University of Glasgow gifted brick scheme reflecting the diverse support and interest in the horse. More recently, the Centre has become the base for the Scottish Performance Horse Clinic which provides a range of innovative diagnostic and

therapeutic modalities for competition horses including: dynamic (exercising) airway endoscopy; radiotelemetric ECG; sensor-based gait analysis; shock wave and stem cell therapies. Led by specialists, Patrick Pollock and David Sutton, it is the only dedicated performance clinic in Scotland, with equipment generously provided by Mark Johnston Racing. Improvements to the centre continue.

The construction of the second stable block was completed in 2009. In addition to doubling the stabling capacity, the new block provides custom designed accommodation to treat critical care cases in adult horses and neonatal foals as well as a 'laminitis box' filled with tons of sand.

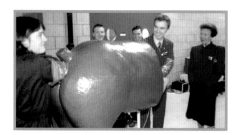

HRH Princess Royal opens the Weipers Centre

The Weipers Centre is staffed by six senior clinicians, three equine veterinary nurses and four grooms. There are four residents training towards eligibility to undertake European College specialist qualifications. As well as providing a 24/7 clinical service to cases referred from throughout Scotland, Northern England and Ireland, the hospital provides year-round clinical training under supervision for senior veterinary students.

2007

Vice Principal Peter Holmes receives OBE.

Tim Greet BVMS 1977

Tim has some great memories of his time as a student appearing as 'Basil Ribbons' and 'David Snow' at the Fresher's Social.[153] He recalls, 'in the 1970s, the Vet School saw its fair share of equine cases'. He describes working with 'the debonair Gordon Baker', a sophisticated Englishman who had established a reputation as a horseman and under whose guidance the Vet School had acquired one of the first flexible fibreoptic units in the UK;

it was promoted extensively. Students were taken on 'scoping expeditions' to local races in Hawick and Penrith.[154] Following a distinguished career in practice, Tim Greet was appointed Honorary Professor of Clinical Equine Studies in the Vet School from 2004 to 2009[155] and was President of the British Equine Veterinary Association in 2000 and President of the British Veterinary Association 2003/2004.

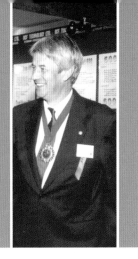

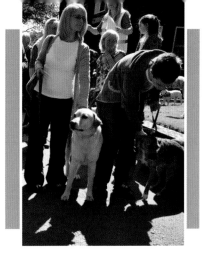

Doggy Dawdle

New small animal hospital - big campaign

In 1998, it was agreed that a new small animal hospital was a priority and that upgrading the current facility was not an option. The A1 Project Committee submitted a proposal to Faculty and funds were obtained from the Glasgow Development Agency to provide consultants on business planning and concept. Stuart Carmichael was appointed project leader. Unfortunately there were many obstacles, particularly finding an appropriate site, and progress was slow. Nevertheless, ambitious plans were made to build a brand new referral hospital.

In November 2004 at the Homecoming Weekend to celebrate the fiftieth anniversary of the first veterinary graduates from the University of Glasgow[156] the opportunity arose to formally launch the campaign to raise funds for the new Small Animal Hospital.[157] The capital appeal was launched by the University to raise £5M of the £15M construction costs with the rest of the money being invested by the School and the University. The hospital case load had grown and student numbers had more than doubled since 1954, when the hospital first opened.

Stuart Carmichael and his team, including Ian Ramsey and Geraldine McCullagh visited leading animal hospitals through the world and drew up plans for a centre for veterinary medicine which would challenge current concepts in clinical practice, teaching and research, and pioneer future standards in animal treatment and welfare.[158]

A competition to appoint the design team generated much interest. The Glasgow practice of Davis Duncan, (later to become part of Archial Architects) was appointed. They were aware of the natural beauty of Garscube and designed the building sympathetically to sit within the landscape.

The first of many fund raising events to take place was a Charity Abseil down the University Tower at Gilmorehill. Over 100 intrepid volunteers descended the 177ft tower, including 'Dougie' the campaign mascot (or rather Glasgow vet and campaign supporter Douglas Hutchison in full size dog suit!)[159, 160]

The inaugural 'Doggy Dawdle', a sponsored 5 kilometre or 10 kilometre walk around the grounds of Garscube in 2005, ran for a further five years – rain or shine.[161]

The Small Animal Hospital campaign received enthusiastic support from alumni, animal lovers including school children and Brownies, staff, and students, celebrities and the grateful owners of patients with first-hand experience of the work undertaken at the Vet School. Over 1,400 donors generously contributed to the campaign.

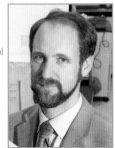

Ian Ramsey

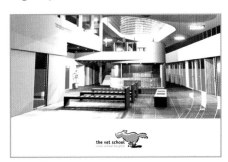

Architect's impression of reception area

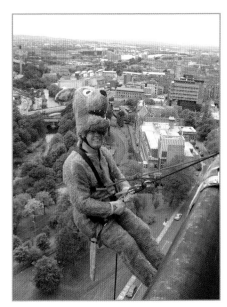

Douglas Hutchison

The SAH workforce is highly qualified and includes fourteen internationally recognised specialists who hold more than forty diplomas and higher degrees between them. Each service is led by at least one specialist. There are also seventeen residents who are training to be specialists and six interns. A recently expanded nursing team includes three senior nurses, eight specialised nurses, sixteen support nurses. There are two radiographers and nine assistant staff. In addition there are forty senior clinical students on rotation at various times during the year.

Any small animal with any problem is seen at any time, when they have been referred from a veterinary surgeon. Patients are initially assigned to particular specialists in areas such as surgery (soft tissue or orthopaedics), neurology, oncology, general medicine, cardiology, ophthalmology or wellness. When they are admitted to the hospital, specialists in anaesthesia and diagnostic imaging are often also involved in the care of the patient.

Clare Knottenbelt is Professor of Small Animal Medicine and Oncology, Clinical Director of the Small Animal Hospital and Head of Small Animal Clinical Sciences.

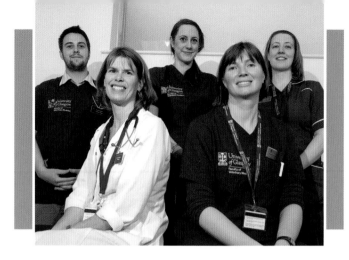

Oncology team 2012

The new Small Animal Hospital opens

After more than ten years in the planning and fundraising, and two years of construction, the new Small Animal Hospital opened for business on 9 September 2009 amid a flurry of media activity. It was worth the wait. Robert Brown, MSP, welcomed the opening in the Scottish Parliament where it was noted as a world class facility for the West of Scotland and the UK as a whole. The building was officially opened by Cabinet Secretary for Finance and Sustainable Growth, John Swinney MSP on 6 July 2010. Guests were greeted by the Veterinary School pipe band, Euan Laidlaw (GUVMA president) and John Marshall, equine surgeon. The new Principal of the University, Professor Anton Muscatelli, in his welcoming address highlighted the Faculty's achievements and paid tribute to the Small Animal Hospital for the outstanding benefits it would bring to patients, their owners, and the staff and students.[162, 163]

The Small Animal Hospital's sophisticated facilities include thirteen consulting rooms, a diagnostic imaging suite complete with MRI and CT scanners, an endoscopy suite, a radioactive iodine unit for treating cats wth hyperthyroidism, a unique pain and rehabilitation centre incorporating a hydrotherapy pool and treadmill together with a physiotherapy suite, state of the art operating theatres, complete with cameras to allow remote viewing of procedures.

The centre for comparative oncology offers a wide range of treatments for most types of cancers in small animals including radiotherapy by a linear accelerator.

Regarded as an architectural landmark, the Small Animal Hospital was named Scotland's best new building, 'a highly complex work of architecture', winning the prestigious Andrew Doolan Prize awarded by the Royal Incorporation of Architects in Scotland, and the Supreme Award from the Glasgow Institute of Architects and in addition won first place in the British Veterinary Association Practice Design Awards in 2011. The building is sensitive and complementary to its environment. It is eco-friendly with a sloping grass roof within which sits an innovative 'crystal' cupola that provides natural light within the building and can be lit with different colours at night. The natural look of the new Hospital is completed with a wall of stone-filled gabion baskets.[164]

Professor Stuart Reid (the Dean at that time) stated, 'The new hospital will allow the vets of tomorrow to learn in the most advanced surroundings, allying the first class building with access to some of the best specialist vets in their field. As a training aid it is unsurpassed'.[165]

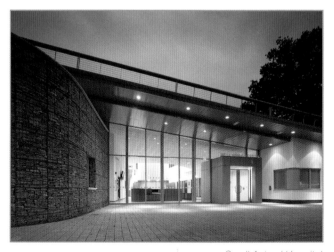

Small Animal Hospital

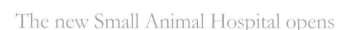

2008

Joint top of all accredited veterinary schools in the RAE.

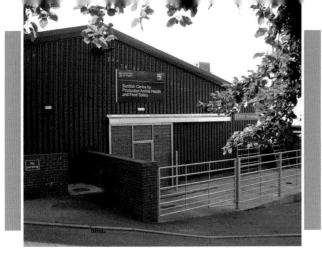

The Scottish Centre for Production Animal Health and Food Safety

The Scottish Centre for Production Animal Health and Food Safety

In 2009 work began on a new farm animal facility, under the guidance of David Logue. The Centre, which was opened in November 2010, is based in the Galloway building, named after the Scotbeef Ltd entrepreneur and philanthropist, Ian Galloway, CBE who provided funding. The construction costs of the new facility were £2M. The Galloway building is linked to the old 'byres', providing flexible and functional accommodation for clinical and veterinary public health teaching at undergraduate and postgraduate level. The 'byres' were refurbished to create seminar and laboratory space, pharmacy facilities, offices, changing areas and stockpersons' accommodation. The buildings are linked by an internal corridor with a bio-zone for boot and hand washing.

The Centre offers a unique service for practitioners and producers throughout Scotland and Northern England. This can involve admission of production animals (cattle, sheep, pigs and camelids) referred by practices for further clinical investigation, diagnosis and treatment, thus meeting the demands of the Scottish Government's initiative to improve animal health and welfare. There is a wealth of expertise available and further investigations may involve the collaboration of colleagues in pathology and farm production record analyses aided by the epidemiology group. In addition visits can be made to farms and processor plants where appropriate. The Centre also includes isolation facilities for animals of higher health status with a view to returning them to their farm after treatment. There is no doubt that this production animal facility is a vast improvement of what was before despite the tears being shed when 'the byres' were flattened!

David Logue officially retired from his position as Professor of Food Animal Disease in 2011. David joined the University from Scottish Agricultural Colleges in 2005.

Through his expertise and office in Scottish BVA, he has had a huge influence on veterinary public policy in Scotland.

The Scottish Centre for Production Animal Health and Food Safety (SCPAHFS) is well staffed with clinical academics, teaching and research academics, clinicians, residents and interns and has a large number of associated staff in the research institutes of the College of Medical, Veterinary and Life Sciences. There are currently three Diplomates of the European College of Bovine Health Management (ECBHM) and two Diplomates of the European College of Veterinary Public Health (ECVPH) with one resident each preparing for examination for their European exams. Staff in the SCPAHFS conduct first opinion clinical work in neighbouring practices and provide a specialist referral service in bovine health management, investigating herd problems such as lameness, mastitis and infertility. The SCPAHFS is heavily involved in undergraduate teaching and makes use of clinical cases referred from surrounding practices as well as the first opinion opportunities afforded by our local practices to train students in the day-one competencies expected of them on graduation. Research is an important activity for most of the staff in the SCPAHFS and its research associates are drawn from the School as well as the Institute for Infection, Immunity and Inflammation and from the Institute of Biodiversity, Animal Health and Comparative Medicine.

The combined group has research strengths in ruminant clinical practice, animal welfare, quantification of disease risk, epidemiology, mathematical modelling, genetics, proteomics and parasitology. Major research themes include the development of evidence based approaches to risk management for livestock diseases, proteomic approaches to identification of disease markers, breeding for resistance to parasitic diseases in farm animals, development of targeted selective treatments for nematode parasites of sheep and cattle, hypothalamic control of reproduction in sheep and cattle, and metabolic diseases of ruminants. The SCPAHFS is within the Division of Large Animal Clinical Sciences and Public Health, led by Professor Dominic Mellor, and the Director of the SCPAHFS is Professor Nick Jonsson.

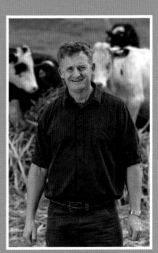

Nick Jonsson

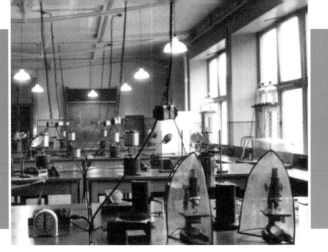

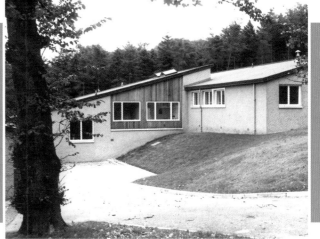

The Research Environment

The old College at Buccleuch Street provided remarkably extensive laboratory space which, considering the poor quality of the fabric of the building, was used to good effect for research, particularly in physiology, parasitology, pathology and microbiology.

Although the original McCall building at Garscube was not designed primarily for research, it did provide some laboratory space for haematology, clinical chemistry, pathology and parasitology. From the 1960s, as a result of the rapidly increasing scientific and commercial success from discoveries at the School, major funding was obtained that enabled construction of research laboratories.

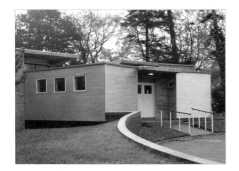

Old Equine Centre

Wellcome/MRC laboratories for experimental parasitology

In the early 1960s following the success of the 'Dictol' vaccine, an application was made to the Wellcome Trust for funds to construct new parasitology laboratories. Unbeknown to the vets, at the same time Adrian Hopkins of the University's Department of Zoology had also submitted an application for new facilities. The Wellcome Trust agreed to fund a single building, the Wellcome Laboratories for Experimental Parasitology at Garscube campus, which were opened in 1964. The ground floor was occupied by a group of parasitologists from Gilmorehill led by Adrian Hopkins, and had an animal house. The upper floor accommodated the veterinary parasitologists including George Urquhart, Jimmy Armour and Frank Jennings. Initially Bill Jarrett, who at that time was Professor of Experimental Veterinary Medicine, was also located in the building, before he was appointed to the Chair of Veterinary Pathology and moved into the Phase I Building in 1969. Later extensions were made to the original structure with funding which had been awarded from various sources to George Urquhart and Ellen Jarrett. These labs were the centre of activity of the Veterinary School's outstanding work in veterinary parasitology for the next fifty years.

The Wellcome Surgical Institute

With the incorporation of the Veterinary School into the Faculty of Medicine, fruitful collaborations in research continued, particularly in veterinary surgery. There was a close association with the department of surgery in Glasgow Royal Infirmary. A small space in the Veterinary Hospital was found for surgeons to undertake work on the human heart lung machine. Following a visit by Sir Henry Dale of the Wellcome Trust, it was decided that support should be given to a surgical research institute to serve both medical and veterinary interests. The Wellcome Surgical Institute facilities included kennel accommodation, an operating theatre, laboratories and observation rooms. The unit was inaugurated by Sir Henry Dale in 1960. It was expanded and extended in 1963 with further grants from the Wellcome Trust. A development fostered by the Wellcome Surgical Institute was the development of the small animal MRI unit which was opened in 2004.

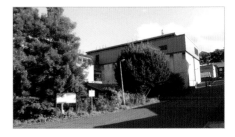

Wellcome Surgical Institute

2008

Professor James McCall Memorial Lecture established.

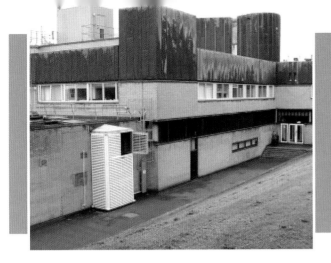

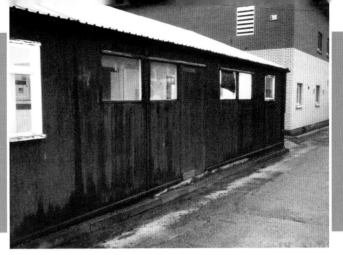

The pre- and para-clinical building (Phase I) at Garscube

The transfer of the departments from Buccleuch Street to Garscube began in 1952 with the clinical departments moving to the Veterinary Hospital. However, for the pre-and para-clinical departments the move took much longer and awaited the construction of a building at Garscube. For anatomy and pathology this meant maintaining their facilities at Buccleuch Street until 1969 while for physiology and biochemistry it involved moving into existing structures at Gilmorehill.

For biochemistry there was total assimilation since the powerful Professor of Biochemistry at the University, Norman Davidson believed 'there is no such subject as veterinary biochemistry, only biochemistry'. However, Robert Garry, Professor of Physiology was prepared to provide office, teaching and research space to the Department of Veterinary Physiology and its recently appointed first professor, Bill Mulligan.

It had been hoped to transfer the whole School to Garscube within a decade of 1949 but shortage of money resulted in delayed building works.

The University of Glasgow fared badly in acquiring building grants from the UGC and no funding had been allocated to the Veterinary School for capital projects between 1955 and 1963. However, in 1963 some funding was made available although the proposed accommodation at Garscube was to be phased. A Phase I building was planned as an ultimate home for all but the pathology group which was to be housed ultimately in a separate Phase II building; in the interim it would be accommodated in Phase I.

However, during preparations for the RCVS quinquennial visit in 1970, the University Development Committee decided that it could not accept the Veterinary School's proposals to go ahead with Phase II. Consequently, pathology remained within the Phase I, now the Jarrett building. Staff also submitted plans at that time for a major extension of clinical departments, including a modern small animal hospital and outpatient departments. Again the University did not recommend the proposals to UGC for funding.[166]

After the pathologists and microbiologists moved to the new phase I building in 1968, Mrs Smith's anatomy department remained the sole occupant of Buccleuch Street until her final move in 1969. As there was no room to house anatomy specimens at Garscube, the lecturers had to drive out daily from the city with the skeletons and specimens needed for teaching in the back of their cars, sometimes spotted with horror by fellow peak hour drivers.

The Buccleuch Street site closed its doors and as it had fallen into disrepair was demolished in 1969. The closing-down party was described as the highlight of the year, 'dancing continued into the wee small hours and as the doors finally closed for the last time, a piper's lament was heard and not a dry eye could be seen'.

In the early 1970s money awarded by the Northumberland Committee, which usually provided only research funding, was used to build extensions to the Phase I building. These included accommodation for the Department of Veterinary Pharmacology and storage facilities for Veterinary Anatomy. In addition this source funded a new two-storey refectory, Surgery offices, a large animal operating theatre and a horse accommodation unit which were constructed opposite the Hospital Building. Alterations to the layout of the Medicine Department floor and improvements to the cattle accommodation were also made.[167]

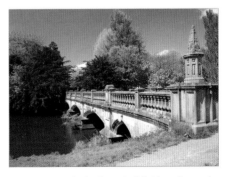

Lady Campbell Bridge, Garscube

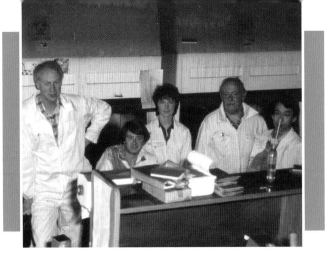

Clearing up following fire 1981

Research in the Phase I building

Initially the Phase I Building was designed to include laboratories for research in bacteriology, physiology, biochemistry, pathology and virology, which were staffed by those who had come from Buccleuch Street together with the hospital pathologists and the feline leukaemia virus group who worked in the small Pfizer Building at Garscube. Subsequent extensions and refurbishments to the main structure provided space for pharmacology as well as an electron microscopy suite. An attached new red brick building of six laboratories for pathology research was provided by funding to Bill Jarrett from the MacRobert Trust.

A major fire occurred in the Phase I Building on the evening of 28 May 1981. The fire destroyed a part of the building which housed mainly the bacteriology and virology laboratories. In addition to water damage, there was a huge loss of equipment, especially high quality pathology microscopes, from the smoke generated by burning plastics. The media reported horror stories of anthrax and radioactivity but in fact these materials had been stored safely. Fortunately, many irreplaceable bacteria, viruses and cell culture lines were stored in liquid nitrogen and remained viable. The insurance assessor was on site the following morning.

James Willison of the Works Department and John Roberts, the Clerk to the Faculty, orchestrated a remarkable and complicated clean-up operation. Although the fire caused much disruption to research and teaching over the succeeding twelve months when temporary accommodation had to be erected in the car park, the recompense from the University's insurance company allowed significant improvements to be made to the laboratories during reinstatement. Refurbishments have continued to be made to the building over the years so that it still provides first-class facilities to its users.

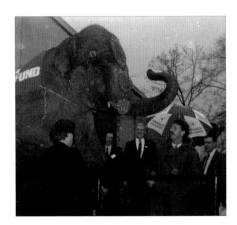

Ian Botham

The Leukaemia Research Fund Virus Centre

The Centre is housed in the two-storey Ian Botham Building adjacent to the MacRobert Trust laboratory block. Funding for the building came from Botham's Hannibal Trek and the laboratories were duly opened by Ian Botham in 1988 with a live elephant and a jazz band in attendance! The former England international cricketer began fundraising in support of leukaemia research in 1987 by walking from John O'Groats to Land's End. This was his first charity walk of many, receiving a knighthood for his efforts in 2007.

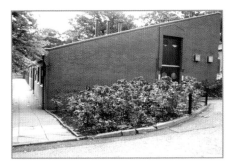

Leukaemia Research Fund Virus Centre

2009

New £2M Scottish Centre for Production Animal Health and Food Safety established at Garscube Campus, replacing 'the byres'.

103

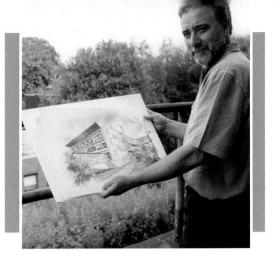

Commercial development facilities

The development of the commercial opportunities emanating from the School's research programme has been an enduring part of the School's history. Key to these developments have been very close and influential links with the Scottish Development Agencies and in particular, Glasgow Development Agency (Margaret McGarry), Dunbartonshire Development Agency (David Macauley), the Scottish Development Agency/ Scottish Enterprise, Glasgow Chamber of Commerce,

and with Central Government, the Department of Trade and Industry and with the European Community such as the European Regional Development Fund. These contacts facilitated the attraction of significant funding (£3.2M) for infrastructure, staff, haematology diagnostics, information and communication technology, database construction and interrogation. The planning for these developments was greatly assisted by the valuable financial advice of Graham Paterson, Director of Glasgow University Holdings Ltd.

Jim Neil with plans for Henry Wellcome building 2002

The Henry Wellcome Building for Comparative Medical Sciences

The Institute of Comparative Medicine was conceived in 1992 as a virtual centre to bring together research across various disciplines in the School's tradition of comparative and interdisciplinary medicine. The idea was transformed with the major award of over £8M from the Wellcome Trust's Science Research Investment Fund in 2001 to allow the beginning of the construction of this new research centre to form the centrepiece of the Institute. Additional funding of £1.7M was obtained from the University of Glasgow.

This impressive building was designed by the Glasgow architects, NJSR Horspool.[168] It comprises a four-storey building which elegantly links the Urquhart and Jarrett buildings with two glazed bridges and has a three-storey high open atrium allowing glimpses of all floors. Staff watched as an extension to the Wellcome Parasitology Building was razed to the ground in less than an hour to make way for the new construction.

There are three storeys of laboratories and offices, topped by a roof-top resource centre which has wonderful views across to the Campsie Fells and beyond, and includes an open air terrace. The Henry Wellcome Building for Comparative Medical Sciences (winner of the Glasgow Institute of Architects Design Award 2005), was officially opened in 2005 by the Chairman of the Wellcome Trust Committee Sir Dominic Cadbury with Sir James Black also in attendance.[169]

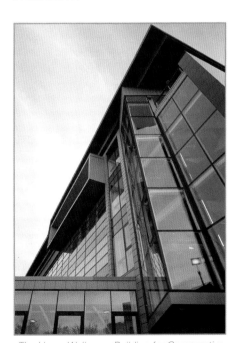

The Henry Wellcome Building for Comparative Medical Sciences

Looking to the future

The Centre for Virus Research

This major infrastructure complex for research will be completed at the School by 2014. The £20M building, to replace the joint University-MRC Institute of Virology currently at Church Street, will house the largest centre in the UK for basic research on viruses, with around 200 members of staff. It will be joined to the Henry Wellcome Building on a site between that building and the Wellcome Surgical Institute. The architects for the project are Sheppard Robson. A very significant part of the remit of the planners is to enhance the surrounding environment which will make a fundamental improvement to the whole School.

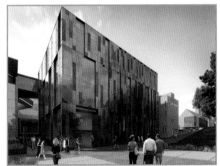

Architects' impression of the Centre for Virus Research

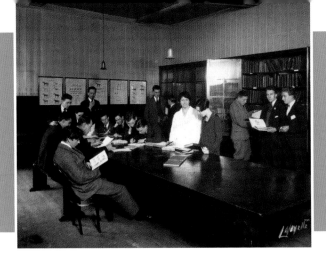

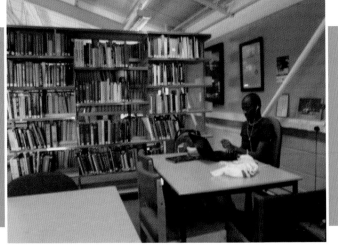

Teaching and student areas

Lecture facilities and practical classes

At the College in Buccleuch Street there was only one lecture theatre and many of the lectures were given in the departmental laboratories. After amalgamation with the University, changes were afoot with the move of the clinical departments to Garscube in 1952. Lectures and practical classes in physics, chemistry, botany, zoology, biochemistry and physiology were held at the main University campus.

The move to Garscube provided greatly improved lecture rooms and clinical facilities for the clinical departments. The lectures centred round the 'Assembly Hall' now the McCall lecture theatre, which was the focus of activities not just for lectures but for staff meetings and social events. There were other smaller lecture rooms on the top and bottom floors of the main building. None of the lecture rooms were 'banked' and students used chairs with flap-down writing boards (which made an almighty clatter when students fell asleep in them!) Another key feature of the new facilities at Garscube and which was later significantly expanded were the post mortem room and large animal demonstration theatre.

Following the construction in 1969 of the Pre-and Para-Clinical Building (Phase I Building) greatly improved teaching facilities were provided for the Anatomy Department with a large dissection laboratory, an adjoining lecture theatre and a large teaching laboratory for histology and laboratory-based para-clinical subjects. However veterinary physiology and biochemistry continued to be taught at Gilmorehill in the Boyd Orr Building.
Over the next forty years the teaching facilities have been continually improved in line with the increasing numbers of undergraduates, the requirements and recommendations of the RCVS quinquennial visitations, and last but not least the availability of suitable funding. Teaching facilities for all parts of the undergraduate course have been improved but perhaps the greatest changes have been in the clinical teaching facilities.

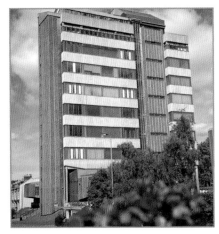

Boyd Orr building

The James Herriot library

At Buccleuch Street the library had been a fairly modest facility on the ground floor and again the move to Garscube provided an opportunity to greatly expand and improve the library provision. From 1952 until 1995 the library was housed on the top floor of the main building and watched over for many decades by the ever-helpful Margaret Postelthwaite.

However as student numbers increased the library became overcrowded and the James Herriot library was built as a third floor on the small animal facility. The former library was converted to a staff amenity area.

The James Herriot library which houses the University of Glasgow's extensive veterinary collection which dates from the 17th century to the present day was opened in 1995. The spacious new library was named after author and graduate Alf Wight in recognition of his services to the veterinary profession. In a letter, Alf Wight said that he regarded this as 'the greatest honour ever bestowed upon him'. The James Herriot Library was opened by his son Jim Wight, himself a Glasgow graduate of 1966. Sadly this was on the day following his father's death on 23 February 1995.[170]

2010
Official opening of the multi award winning new Small Animal Hospital.

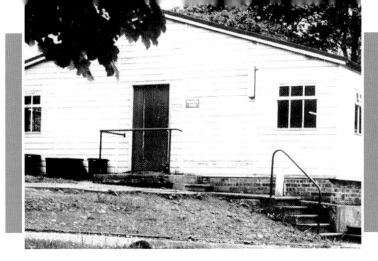
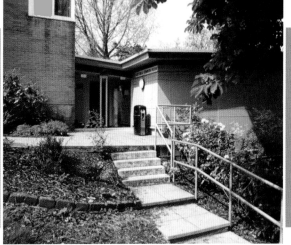

The GUVMA Hut

With the amalgamation of the Veterinary College
and the University of Glasgow, the old Glasgow
Veterinary Medical Association became the
Glasgow University Medical Association
(GUVMA), but students still had to use the old
common room facilities at Buccleuch Street.
With the evacuation of Buccleuch Street,
it was necessary to provide new facilities.[171]
With funding from the Carnegie Trust and
the centenary appeal, Weipers suggested a
building 'made from attractive African hardwood
incorporating some of the features of the
recreation pavilion which could occupy a site
overlooking the river, …often seen in chalet
buildings in Switzerland'.[172] Alas this dream was
never realised and a more utilitarian wooden
shed was constructed. Many students will
remember (or not!) fun occasions held within.
Although fragile in appearance, it was robust
in practice. The new GUVMA Common Room
opened in 1996 to replace the old GUVMA hut,
however it has been demolished as part of the
GLASS project.[173]

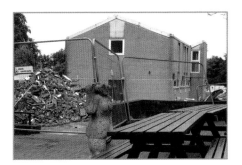

Building demolition begins 2012

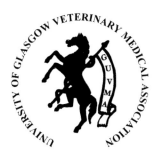
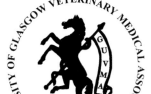

The GLASS project

The Garscube Learning and Social Space
(GLASS) project is a new major building
proposal for the Garscube campus. Its aim
is to provide a learning and social hub for the
whole campus. It will involve a new build on
the site of the front of the former small animal
hospital to house a cafe and social space
with a linked flexible study and learning area.
The space in the former hospital behind the
new building will be converted into a series
of tutorial and study rooms. The Campbell,
Stewart and large animal surgery buildings
and the Isolation Unit will all be demolished.
The project also involves a proposal to
enhance the McCall and Animal Health
Teaching Complex lecture theatres.

In addition, the University proposes to
implement a 'campus development' project
to improve the landscape and infrastructure of
the estate. This project is being taken forward
alongside the GLASS project and the MRC
Centre for Virus Research building.

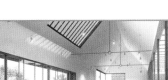
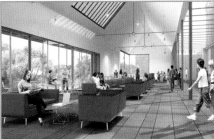
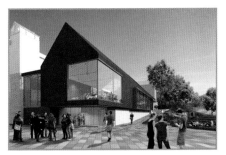

Architects' impression of GLASS project

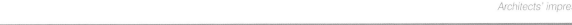

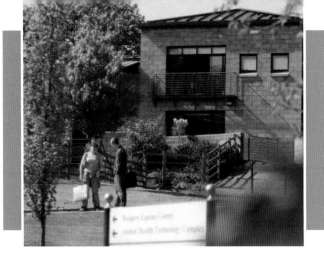
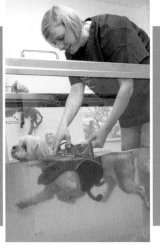
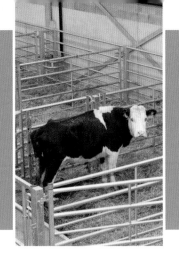

Students outside Weipers Centre   Small Animal Hospital   SCPAHFS

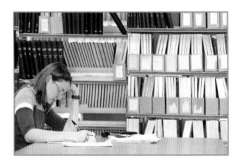

Conclusions

The development of Garscube has been a fascinating journey and an outstanding confirmation of the wisdom of William Weipers' one-site vision of a veterinary science centre in close proximity to the main campus with its medical and science faculties, and the agriculture complex of Cochno.

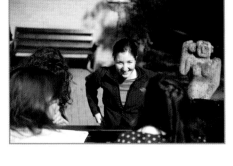

Sixty years ago the newly built Veterinary Hospital sat in splendid isolation surrounded by pleasant wooded parkland. Over the years, the Garscube campus has filled up, with extensions to the original Hospital building and then many additions, together with the re-siting of the Beatson Institute for Cancer Research and the University's sports complex in the grounds. Much of the development of the School is a product of self-reliance, funded through the success of our research and teaching, and the respect and appreciation of the local and the wider veterinary community.

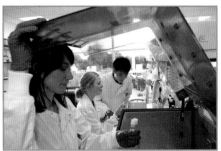

Though it is the staff and students of Glasgow Veterinary School that make the place so unique, the development of facilities over recent years has greatly enhanced the student and staff experience. This is reflected not only in the clinical buildings, including the award winning Small Animal Hospital, the Weipers Centre for Equine Welfare and the Scottish Centre for Production Animal Health and Food Safety, but also in the research buildings including the Henry Wellcome building. This will be strengthened further with the building of the MRC Centre for Virus Research in the near future.

Our students have long had a reputation of being a sociable bunch, a most important requisite of a veterinary surgeon. The GUVMA huts old and new have been focal to many high spirited student events. With the imminent construction of the new social area as part of the GLASS project, and the state of the art clinical and teaching facilities, many further cohorts of students are destined to continue the 'work hard, play hard' ethos of the Glasgow Veterinary School.

2010
Faculty translated from 'Faculty of Veterinary Medicine' to 'School of Veterinary Medicine' within the College of Medical, Veterinary and Life Science

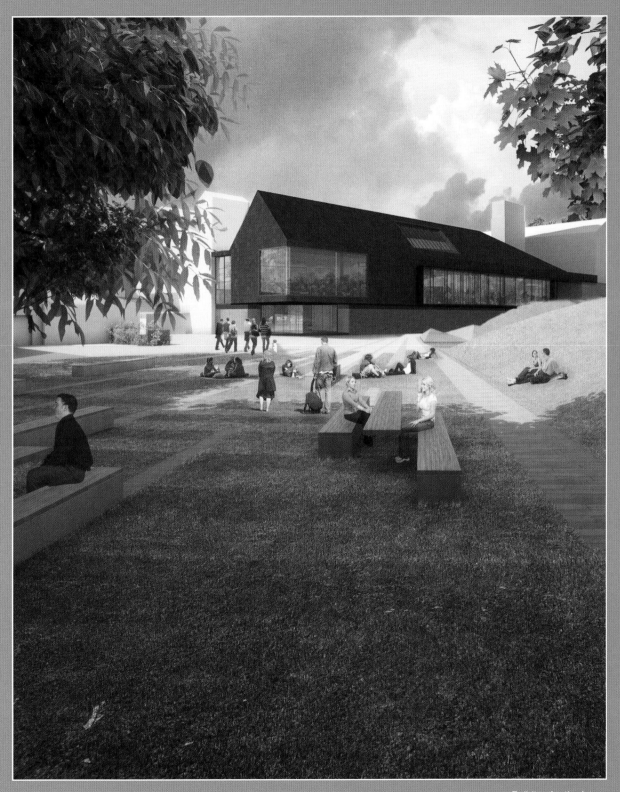

Building for the future

Chapter Six

Glasgow Vets Overseas

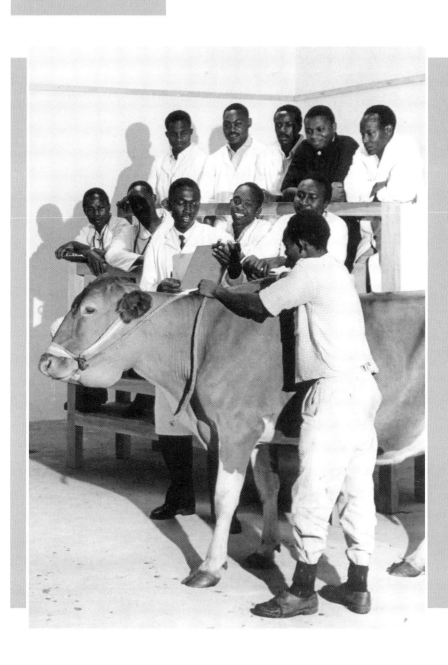

Vets Overseas

Throughout the years, Glasgow vets and alumni have forged strong links in many parts of the world, especially in Africa, developing veterinary services, building veterinary schools, establishing international research centres and research networks and contributing to animal and human health and welfare.

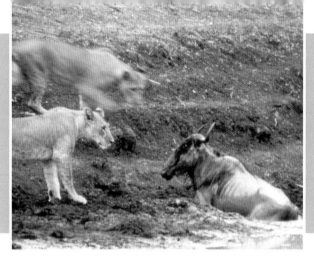

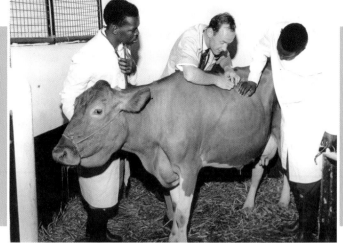

Tsavo River

Douglas McEwan teaching in Nairobi, 1950s

Early days

The University of Glasgow and Scotland have had enduring collaborations with Africa since the days of David Livingstone, who not only contributed to the exploration of this vast continent, but also to our understanding of the contagia of man and animals, in particular the dreaded 'Tsetse Fly Disease'. Livingstone recognised that his oxen and horses became sick when bitten by tsetse flies and he even suggested successful treatments in a letter to the British Medical Journal in 1858 although the trypanosome parasite transmitted by the tsetse fly was not identified until 1900 by another Scot, David Bruce. Later work in 1910 in Uganda by Muriel Robertson, an Arts graduate from Glasgow University who became engrossed with protozoan research, described for the first time the parasite's life cycle in the tsetse fly and in infected animals.

Meanwhile back in Glasgow, of James McCall's five sons who became vets, two of them could not attend his funeral in 1915 because they were working in South Africa and Nyasaland.

Veterinary services and research in West Africa

In the 1930s -1950s there were many Glasgow vets working across Africa, especially in West Africa, in the provision of veterinary services and in veterinary research where they made major contributions. For example in Nigeria, the Federal Director of Veterinary Services in the 1950s was Roy Marshall, a 1930s graduate while the Regional Director of Veterinary Services in Eastern Nigeria and Cameroon were John McCulloch (early 1950s) followed by Ian Macfarlane, both of whom were 1940s graduates of Glasgow. From the 1950s era, Ross Brewster ran the veterinary service in the capital, Lagos and Forrest Laing and John Smith worked in the Northern Region.
Bill Ferguson (1950s graduate) was the first to describe the potential of the native dwarf cattle (muturu) to survive and thrive in areas endemic for trypanosomiasis in Southern Nigeria. John McCulloch who moved to the Northern Province in 1955 carried out pioneering control of tsetse fly habitats using aerial spraying with insecticide.

The Federal Research Centre at Vom, Nigeria was involved in animal production research and included a very active parasitology group whose membership included John Ross and James Armour who described for the first time inherited resistance to intestinal helminths in the progeny of selected bulls and seasonal hypobiosis (arrested development) of gastric nematodes in cattle.

At the same laboratories, the production of viral and bacterial vaccines for cattle throughout West Africa was a major feature and Alan McLeod was senior member of the production and testing team.

In the late 1940s and 1950s rinderpest was controlled in Nigeria and other West African countries with a vaccine prepared from infected goat spleens and used to protect Zebu cattle and a lapanised vaccine to protect the much more susceptible N'Dama cattle which are popular, particularly in the Western Region because of their trypanotolerance.

In 1949 Donald Hamilton was the veterinary officer in The Gambia at the time of the ill-fated Gambia egg scheme thought up by Stafford Cripps, a Minister in the post war Atlee Government. Donald was responsible for the reports which highlighted the massive mortality due to Newcastle disease in the imported British poultry breeds lacking in immunity to the disease.

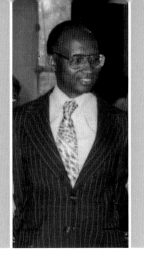

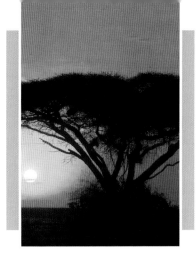

As a result of the Glasgow influence, numerous local West Africans came to study veterinary medicine at Glasgow. Among them were Sir Dawda Jawara who eventually entered politics and was President of Gambia for twenty seven years, and Protus Atang from the Cameroons who after serving as a veterinary officer in Nigeria moved to Kenya, thence to become Director General of OAU/IBAR (Organisation of African Unity/Interafrican Bureau of Animal Resources). Later Glasgow also developed strong links in South America (Argentina, Paraguay, Brazil and Ecuador), the Middle East especially Iraq, and the West Indies where Sir William Weipers had strong interests. All of these connections brought a stream of students to Glasgow, particularly at postgraduate level.

Veterinary Schools in East Africa: 1963 and onwards

Sir William Weipers' interest in veterinary education extended overseas. He became involved with the Food and Agriculture Organisation (FAO) and the World Health Organisation (WHO), joining an expert panel which was designed to study a curriculum that could be adapted by veterinary schools in developing countries. At this time, in the early 1960s, 'the wind of change' was sweeping across Africa and many independent states were emerging.

A major challenge to many of these nations was that their economies were based largely on livestock and agriculture, and were under massive threat from infectious diseases of animals and of man. In 1961, Sir Thomas Dalling, a Senior Veterinary Consultant at FAO, and former lecturer at the College, stated that 5000 vets were needed in Africa but only 2000 existed for the whole continent, of which1500 were in Egypt and 500 were spread over the rest of Africa; ninety percent were expatriates.

At the same time, George Urquhart who had gone to Kenya in the late 1950s to become head of parasitology at the East African Veterinary Research Organisation (EAVRO) at Muguga, advised that while there were only two local professionally qualified veterinary surgeons in Kenya, there was a fledgling veterinary school in Nairobi, part of The University College Nairobi within The University of East Africa, founded in 1962. In addition, there were many highly capable animal health paraveterinary Diplomats (Kenyans, Ugandans, and Tanzanians) from The University of Makerere, Uganda.

Encouraged by Weipers, in 1960 Ian McIntyre went to New York, and presented a proposal that was accepted by the Rockefeller Foundation. This meeting established a relationship that was to last for over forty years. Funded by the Foundation, a masterplan was prepared in consultation with the University of East Africa; in October 1963, some forty selected animal health Diplomates from Makerere would undergo an intensive fortyeight week clinically-led interdisciplinary course, popularly known as the 'conversion course', upgrading them to internationally recognised degree status. There would be an extra term for those who failed the final examination first time.

Conversion Course, Vet School Kabete, 1964

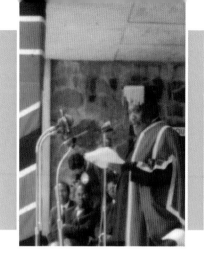
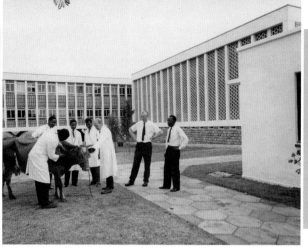
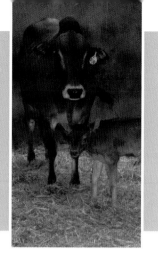

Graduation, President Kenyatta 1964 | Ian McIntyrre, Peter Nderito and Hugh Pirie, Nairobi 1966 | Boran surrogate mother, N'Dama calf

In August 1963 a team from Glasgow led by Ian McIntyre and including Bill Jarrett, George Urquhart, Bill Martin and families, travelled to Kenya. They were accompanied by several young veterinary members of staff including Max Murray, Douglas McEwan and Ian Glen, technical staff and secretaries totalling nearly forty in the first wave.

Ian McIntyre quickly integrated this team with personnel from the fledgling Veterinary School at the Kabete and Chiromo campuses, EAVRO at Muguga, including the eminent Walter Plowright who developed the first effective rinderpest vaccine, the Government Veterinary Laboratories and the Wellcome Research Laboratories at Kabete and visiting staff from veterinary schools in Giessen, Fort Collins and Oslo.

In November 1964, the Veterinary Diplomates were presented by Ian McIntyre to the Chancellor, Jomo Kenyatta, who had become the first President of Kenya in 1963, to President Julius Nyerere of Tanzania, to the Vice-President of Uganda and to Malcolm MacDonald, the British High Commissioner. These were some of the first graduates of the University College Nairobi (previously students had received graduate status from Universities outwith Africa). These graduates subsequently came to occupy many of the most senior veterinary positions throughout Africa.

Concurrently, a five year curriculum was embedded into the Veterinary School. The format for this, as with the conversion course, was clinically driven. The Veterinary School became a Faculty of the University College Nairobi, in the University of East Africa in 1965, with Ian McIntyre as founding Dean, a post he held for three and a half years on secondment from Glasgow. Over this period, the limited facilities at Kabete were complemented by new state of the art technology and research facilities funded by the US Agency for International Development.

In 1964 and 1965, a second wave of personnel arrived including Jim Duncan, Hugh Miller, Tom Miller, Craig Sharp, George Crighton, Hugh and Myrtle Pirie, Ted Fisher, Frank Jennings and family, Jimmy Campbell and family, Tom Douglas and family and several of the first wave returned to their duties in Glasgow. Over the next decade, more than a hundred members of staff from Glasgow with their families rotated through Nairobi Veterinary School.

Many of the lessons learned during the 'conversion course years' were taken back to Glasgow and unquestionably contributed to its future academic strategy and research success. The contribution of Glasgow University was officially described at the time as 'the biggest effort so far made by a British University in African higher education'.

Later in the decade when the East African Confederation broke up, McIntyre and colleagues were involved in progressing the new veterinary schools at Makerere, Uganda and Sokoine, Tanzania, and advising on the curriculum at Lusaka, Zambia and Harare, Zimbabwe. In 1979 Peter Holmes and others from Glasgow assisted in the development of the Ethiopian Veterinary School at Debre Zeit. The founding Dean was the highly effective Feseha Gabreab and he developed the School into one of the finest in Africa. He received an honorary degree from the University of Glasgow in 2001. The longstanding relationship between the Ethiopian Veterinary School and Glasgow also fostered the development of donkey clinics in Ethiopia funded by the UK's Donkey Sanctuary and closely involved Jim Duncan and Stuart Reid.

During Glasgow's involvement in the establishment of the Nairobi Veterinary School a variety of research programmes were initiated on diseases affecting domestic animals as well as wildlife. Ground breaking studies were carried out by Bill Jarrett, George Crighton and Hugh Pirie on the life cycle and kinetics of replication of the protozoan parasite, *Theileria parva*, the cause of East Coast Fever, a widespread and lethal tick-borne disease of cattle, work that was seminal to future vaccination development programmes by Matt Cunningham.

2010
Official opening of the Scottish Centre for Production Animal Health and Food Safety.

113

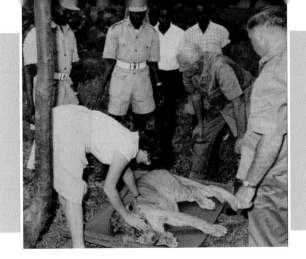
Heather Campbell with Tiva, 1964

Several novel conditions were encountered such as papillomas in association with vulvo-cutaneous carcinomas in cattle, transmissible venereal tumour in dogs and *Spirocerca lupi* in dogs, a putative cause of oesophageal sarcomas, all relevant to future cancer research. Another rewarding discovery was finding that muscular dystrophy was common in several species of antelope, most importantly the rare Hunter's antelope. This condition is a treatable vitamin E/selenium deficiency that occurs also in cattle in Scotland.

The lack of qualified veterinary surgeons in Kenya in the early 1960s was matched by the lack of medical doctors. In 1964, Ian McIntyre made contact with the Medical School at the University of Glasgow and soon afterwards Sir Charles Fleming who was Dean of the Medical Faculty along with Professor William Arthur Mackey and colleagues visited Nairobi on a 'safari' that resulted in the establishment of a medical school there, with a Medical Faculty opening in 1967. The initial funding was from Overseas Development Administration (ODA).

New international research laboratories (1970- 1980s)

International Laboratory for Research on Animal Diseases - Nairobi, Kenya

Seeds sown by the experience in Nairobi Veterinary School germinated into 'blue sky' discussions during the 1960s, often along the banks of the River Kelvin at Garscube. The result was McIntyre and the Glasgow team submitting another concept note to the Rockefeller Foundation in 1969 which was to have a major impact on research in Glasgow and Africa over the next forty years including the establishment of two international research institutes.

Vets in the Wild

The catchment area for the vets of the University of Nairobi encompassed the Nairobi National Park. It was home to wild animals rescued from various unfortunate circumstances or 'unmanageable or unwanted wild animal pets' collected from owners. Heather Campbell (formerly Heather Martin BVMS 1954) who ran the popular small animal clinic for the Faculty of Veterinary Medicine for the University of Nairobi was the veterinary surgeon called upon to treat their ailments. Her husband Bob describes a memorable case of 'A Lion for the Emperor'. In 1964, a young orphaned lion named Tiva - also the name of the river that runs through the northern end of the Tsavo East National Park in Kenya, had been chosen as a gift for the Emperor of Ethiopia, from the President of Kenya, Jomo Kenyatta to cement the good relationship of neighbours. Tiva was placed in a crate and driven to Nairobi Airport for shipment by air to Addis Ababa.

However the crate was not strong enough to hold Tiva and he broke out and leapt off the moving vehicle only to damage his left hind limb in the fall. He was recaptured and returned to his cage at the orphanage before an urgent call was placed to Heather. Together with Sydney Jennings (Professor of Surgery at Glasgow at this time) who was visiting Kenya, she drove to the orphanage to examine a sedated Tiva. He had fractured his femur. It was decided to attend to the break as soon as possible and a suitable pin, one designed for a human, was eventually obtained from the Nairobi Hospital. The next afternoon Tiva was again sedated, hoisted into a Volkswagen pick up and driven to the Small Animal Clinic! Professor Jennings acted as anaesthetist and Sir William Weipers, Heather's former Dean acted as her assistant. The operation went relatively smoothly and he recovered remarkably quickly. Fortunately he was rehomed in Nairobi National Park rather than the Royal establishment at Addis Ababa. [175]

At the same time in Glasgow, a major research commitment to tropical disease, in particular African trypanosomiasis in both animals and man, evolved and continues to the present time. During this time major advances were already taking place in the major viral diseases of domestic livestock, including, rinderpest and foot and mouth disease. The philosophy of the concept note was that an international research effort was needed to tackle the major parasitic diseases of domestic livestock that were holding captive vast areas of the most productive land in Africa. One of these research institutes should be based in East Africa where there was already an infrastructure of parastatal organisations, including the EAVRO and the East African Trypanosomiasis Research Organisation (EATRO). The institute should be staffed by vets and basic scientists. There would be a Glasgow team of a multidisciplinary structure functioning in an interdisciplinary fashion. The key was that these researchers would have direct access to the disease in the field. At the same time, they would have the budget to involve researchers and institutes throughout the world. The Centre would have a Rockefeller–like postdoctoral programme with a long-term strategy of training scientists, importantly to include Africans.

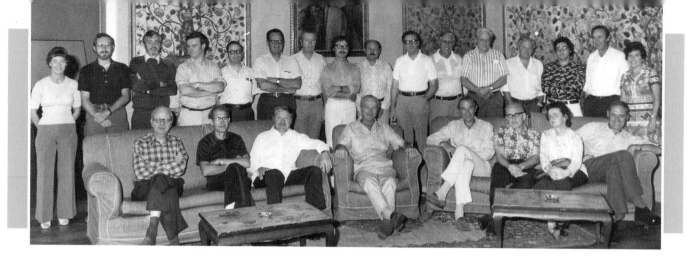

Think-tank meetings were held, mainly at the Rockefeller Conference Centre at the Villa Serbelloni, Bellagio, on Lake Como from the early 1970s, where it was agreed that an institute called the International Laboratory for Research on Animal Diseases (ILRAD) should be established in Nairobi.

The main objectives were to develop effective control measures and novel vaccines for livestock diseases that seriously limited world food production, focusing in the first instance on tsetse–transmitted African trypanosomiasis and tick-borne diseases, particularly East Coast Fever, a virulent form of theileriosis.

ILRAD became one part of a multi-million dollar global agricultural research centre network sponsored by the Consultative Group on International Agricultural Research (CGIAR) conceived by the Rockefeller Foundation in 1968. CGIAR headquarters are located in the World Bank, Washington, DC.

It was widely expected that Ian McIntyre or Bill Jarrett would be appointed Director General. However, McIntyre was heavily committed to another major initiative in The Gambia with the International Trypanotolerance Centre (ITC), West Africa, while Bill Jarrett had other irons in the fire in the fields of virology and cancer research. Professor Jim Henson of the College of Veterinary Medicine at Washington State University was appointed in 1974.

In 1975 Max Murray was appointed ILRAD's first Senior Scientist and he played a key role over the next few years in the recruitment of research personnel, including several from Glasgow including Jack Doyle, who later became Deputy Director General, and Ivan Morrison. Through many shared research grants and shared postgraduates, close links were maintained with Glasgow.

A magnificent, state of the art research institute was officially opened in April 1978 by Daniel Arap Moi, Vice President and subsequently President of Kenya.

ILRAD grew to be one of the leading animal disease research laboratories in the world, having at one time scientists of twentyone nationalities. While the vaccine against trypanosomiasis is still awaited, major advances were achieved in understanding its pathology, pathogenesis, immunology, diagnosis and genetic resistance. Also, ILRAD in collaboration with the International Livestock Centre for Africa (ILCA) (ILCA/ILRAD Trypanotolerance Network), the ITC and Glasgow, carried out some of the most extensive studies ever done on drug control and trypanotolerant livestock. In 1994, ILRAD merged with ILCA, Ethiopia, to form the International Livestock Research Institute (ILRI).

Possibly, ILRAD's greatest success was that it helped stimulate global action on the world's great forgotten exotic diseases of animals and man.

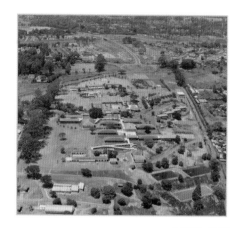

ILRAD, 1978

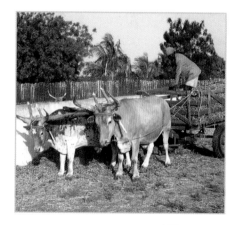

N Dama oxen

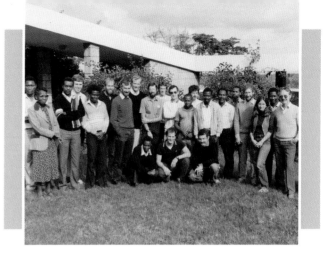

ILRAD, 1984

Max Murray BVMS 1962

'The Glasgow Team' integrated well into the social and academic life of the University in Nairobi, as well as the various Social Clubs key to the infrastructure of Kenya. In 1964 and 1965, Ian McIntyre and Bill Martin participated in the East Africa Safari Car rally. They drove an MG1100, and an Red and Black Mini Cooper S, the first in East Africa. Another consequence of the 'Nairobi' experience is that Glasgow staff to this day are commonly *employed as consultants and advisors, and committees to all the major international organisations involved in worldwide animal and human health e.g. WHO, FAO, OAU/IBAR. An example of our reputation was that we were invited to run a 'Leadership Training Seminar' on Tsetse – Borne Trypanosomiasis organised by FAO/OAU/WHO in collaboration with ILRAD, Nairobi, Kenya: in 1977. The course lasted three weeks and had sixtynine participants from twentyfive African countries.*

The International Trypanotolerance Centre in The Gambia, West Africa

In the early 1970s, as part of an ongoing research programme on African trypanosomiasis at Glasgow, attention was drawn by Sir Dawda Jawara to the indigenous *Bos taurus* breeds of cattle in West and Central Africa which were reputed to possess significant resistance to African trypanosomiasis, termed 'trypanotolerance', and to other important endemic diseases related to ticks and helminths. The N'Dama, the most common breed of this type, is believed to be derived from the Hamitic Longhorn which was first depicted in cave paintings in Africa around 5000 BC and to be the first domestic cattle to settle in Africa. As part of the Glasgow African diaspora, the Rockefeller Foundation funded Glasgow to assess the phenomenon of trypanotolerance. Thus in 1973, Ian McIntyre led a team to The Gambia, where the N'Dama, is predominant.

They were based at the veterinary laboratories at Abuko (Director: Wally N'Dow and Bakary Sanyang, a Senior Animal Health Technician) and at the MRC Research Laboratories (Director: Sir Ian MacGregor).

The preliminary results were promising and an expanded Glasgow team revisited in 1974, and then a resident group led by Keith Murray and Derek Clifford in 1975. Funding was extended by the Rockefeller Foundation in 1976 and beyond. This work drew attention to the potential of N'Dama and other indigenous breeds such as the West African Shorthorn, as well as to local breeds of sheep and goats, as a means of increasing production in the vast tsetse-infested humid and sub-humid areas of Sub-Saharan Africa.

Thus the concept of setting up a centre of excellence in Africa to carry out definitive studies on genetic resistance evolved. Sir Dawda Jawara, through Ian McIntyre with sponsorship from the Rockefeller Foundation organised a conference of eminent scientists, donor agencies and multinational institutes at the Villa Serbelloni, Bellagio in 1981, to consider this proposal. An Enabling Act setting up the ITC in The Gambia was passed by the Gambian Government in 1982. Funding was provided initially by the Gambian Government, the African Development Bank, Rockefeller Foundation, Britain (ODA/DFID), then European Community through ILRAD/ILCA and later Switzerland and Belgium.

Ian McIntyre was appointed first Director General in 1984. Construction of ITC at three sites throughout The Gambia, Kerr Serigne, Keneba and Bansang was completed and opened in 1987.

It was considered by FAO as one of the most innovative and best 'blueprints' for a research field centre in the world. ITC helped to focus world attention on the potential of genetic resistance as a significant weapon for disease control. Glasgow Veterinary School was the catalyst and driving force. Max Murray served as Chairman of the Programme Committee and Member of the Executive. The immunologist Tony Davies was the dynamic Chairman of the ITC Council. Later Peter Holmes served on ITC Council 1996-2006.

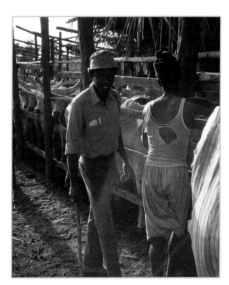

Bakary Sanyang. 1974

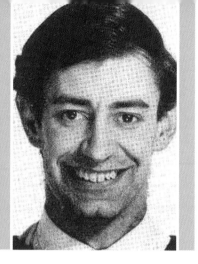
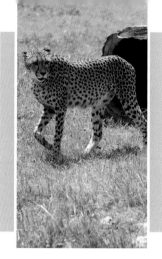

Craig Sharp

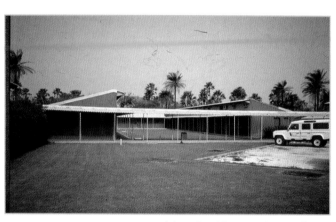

International Trypanotolerance Centre

Trypanosomiasis

The close involvement of Glasgow vets in East Africa in the 1960s stimulated a major interest in the exotic diseases of animals and man that enslave Africa. At the start of the 1970s, George Urquhart and Ian McIntyre and their teams turned their interest to control of tsetse-transmitted trypanosomiasis, a disease that devastates animal and man in an area of Africa larger than the USA. At the same time, at Gilmorehill, Keith Vickerman had recently been appointed to the Zoology Department and was developing a major programme investigating the antigens of the surface coat of the trypanosome with a view to using them for vaccination.

Studies of trypanosome infections began in mice at the Veterinary School and these were quickly followed by the opportunity to conduct studies in cattle when Peter Holmes was seconded to the Institute of Pathobiology in Addis Ababa in 1972.

There it was possible to undertake experimental infections to begin investigations into the pathogenesis of bovine trypanosomiasis and also to start studies on the judicious use of trypanocidal drugs to control trypanosomiasis in oxen used in settlement schemes in lowland areas of Ethiopia heavily infested with tsetse flies.

This programme of research continued in Ethiopia during the 1970s and was considerably extended as improved facilities became available at ILRAD and ITC.

Facilities were developed at the Veterinary School in Glasgow to permit the infection of ruminants with pathogenic trypanosomes and allowing research to be conducted in parallel with studies in Africa. Thus Glasgow became a world centre for trypanosomiasis research from the early 1960s.

In order to maximise these approaches, the Glasgow team became part of an international consortium adopting its well proven strategies for disease control. Using mostly laboratory animals in Glasgow and domestic ruminants in Africa, mainly in The Gambia, Ethiopia and ILRAD, the main pathogenic processes were identified and characterised. This research confirmed that anaemia was the key pathogenic driving force in ruminants; that immunosuppression develops, confirmed in Ethiopia in Zebu cattle often predisposing them to secondary infection or impaired vaccination such as to foot and mouth vaccine; and that there was widespread tissue damage, mainly of the brain and heart, manifested particularly with the tissue invasive *Trypanosoma brucei* subgroup. *T. congolense* and *T. vivax*, the main pathogenic species found in ruminants. They are confined largely to the circulation, and hence anaemia is the dominant pathogenic factor. Infections are also detrimental to reproductive function in both males and females. All of these pathogenic effects of trypanosome infections in ruminants were shown through the work of Eli Katunguka, Jim Parkins, Peter Holmes and others, to be markedly affected by the level of host nutrition and especially protein intake.

2012
The School celebrates 150 years since its foundation in 1862.

117

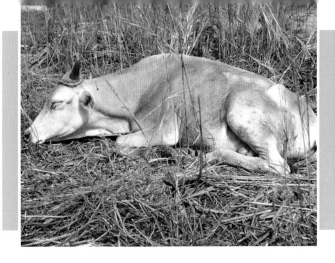

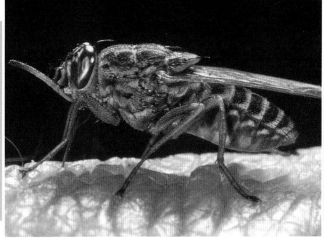

N'Dama cow with sleeping sickness

Tsetse fly feeding

Trypanosomiasis control strategies

Two key pieces of work laid the basis for approaches to disease control in cattle. The first was the measurement of anaemia by packed red cell volume (PCV) and the second was detection of the parasite, both using the same microhaematocrit capillary tube. This point-of-care technology, developed by Glasgow scientists, played a pivotal role in trypanosomiasis diagnosis in evaluating drug control, and the performance of trypanotolerant breeds, in some of the largest livestock development programmes ever undertaken in tsetse-infested Africa. This involved the analysis of massive databases by the joint ILCA/ILRAD Trypanotolerance Network. Established in 1977, the Network had operations in thirteen countries in West, Central and East Africa. This operation confirmed the effectiveness and profitability of drug control and, for the first time, showed the productive potential of trypanotolerant livestock.

Glasgow stimulated a truly international effort involving African villagers, privately owned ranches, government agencies, international organisations, Rockefeller Foundation, international research centres, including ILRAD, ILCA and ITC and pharmaceutical companies, including, May and Baker Ltd. and Hoescht AG.

Control options for trypanosomiasis are limited in man and animals. Tsetse control and eradication has proved costly, complex and is rarely sustainable. A vaccine was not available and is not likely to be in the foreseeable future, because of the capacity of trypanosomes to undergo protective antigen variation. Thus, disease control has been largely dependent on a limited number of drugs developed in the 1950s and 1960s, and on naturally-occurring disease resistance. The research programme of the Glasgow team focussed on achieving improved use of these two control methods.

The use of trypanocidal drugs

Throughout the 1980s joint research between scientists in Glasgow and ILRAD investigated the factors influencing the duration of trypanocidal drug prophylaxis against challenge by drug-susceptible and drug-resistant trypanosomes, the development of new tests for trypanocidal drug-resistance including the use of novel immunoassays for drug detection, and identification of the factors influencing the development of drug-resistance by trypanosomes. Key staff included in this research included Mark Eisler, Douglas Whitelaw, Andrew Peregrine, Keith Sones, and Grace Murilla.

Crucial factors in planning drug control strategies in the field included the level of tsetse risk, the mode of action of drugs available (therapeutic or prophylactic) and the management infrastructure. Where the tsetse risk was low and where there was good management infrastructure, the use of therapeutic drugs were most likely to be considered. However, where the risk was high, the drug of choice would be prophylactic with a duration that could stretch to six months.

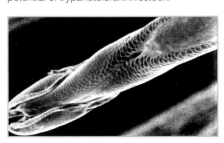

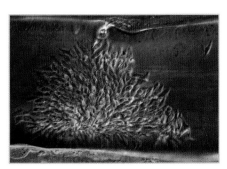

Tsetse proboscis

Trypanosomes injected through proboscis

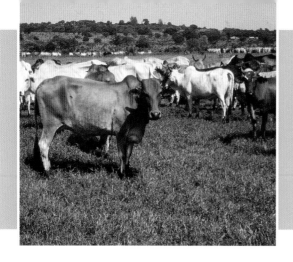
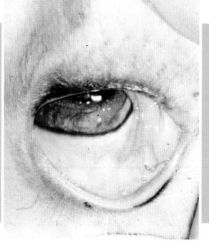
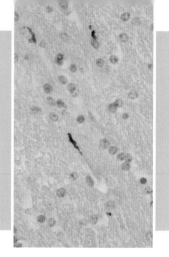

Grade Boran at Mkwaja Ranch   Anaemia due to trypanosomiasis   Histology showing trypanosomes

Glasgow scientists played a significant advisory role in some extensive and comprehensive studies using drug control. For example, in Kilifi Plantations near Mombasa, the dairy ranch was one of the biggest in Africa covering 2,700 hectares and carrying 2,500 animals (*Bos indicus*-Sahiwal /Ayrshire crosses). The control strategy advised and adopted used PCV estimation as the indicator of infection and treatment with the therapeutic trypanocidal drug Berenil. Comprehensive databases of animal health and productivity parameters were maintained and the control strategy recommended proved successful and profitable over a period of twenty years.

A further example of Glasgow's input took place at Mkwaja Ranch Amboni Ltd., Arusha, Tanzania. This was established in 1954 with the intention of supplying the labour force of Amboni Sisal Estates with meat from a herd of 12,000 grade Boran (*Bos indicus*) cattle.

The ranch, of nearly 50,000 hectares, was situated on the north east coast of Tanzania in an area heavily infested with tsetse. Massive efforts were made to control the deadly trypanosomiasis risk. Eradication and control of tsetse and trypanocidal drugs were all deployed over many years without success. In 1973, a rigorous combined prophylactic and chemotherapeutic treatment control strategy was proposed by Glasgow scientists and adopted. Management infrastructure was of the highest standard.

The databases maintained were unique by virtue of their volume and completeness comprising over 20,000 data per trait (1973-1982), yielding matching animal health, trypanocidal drug treatment, and composite animal productivity indices. Over the ten year period, the consequence was that acceptable levels of productivity and profit were attained. The productivity achieved at Mkwaja was close to that of Boran reared in tsetse-free conditions in ranches in Kenya.

The vast majority of cattle in Sub-Saharan Africa are kept by smallholders with two to four animals, sometimes mixed in a collective herd. In such situations the rigorous management, described previously at Kilifi and Mkwaja, was not an option. A study was carried out at Muhaka on the Kenyan coast. It is a village area of some 100 km^2 and is an area of medium tsetse risk. There were some 700 East African Zebu cattle in seventeen village herds belonging to thirtyone owners. Trypanosomiasis was known to be the main disease.

The strategy adopted was to treat the cattle three times per year with Samorin. In addition, any individual animal detected as parasitaemic or showing clinical signs was inoculated with Berenil. Over the four year study, the increase in productivity computed on the basis of key production parameters, including lactation, was over 30 percent. The resultant economic benefit covered veterinary services and drug cost as the money was in the milk.

Consequently, exotic dairy cow genes were successfully introduced by artificial insemination into this area by the Kenyan Government and the programme was extended throughout the Coast Province and into Tanzania.

At the time, these results reported in the late 1970s and 1980s had major consequences in confirming the economic viability of drug control of Bovine African Trypanosomiasis to livestock owners and to the pharmaceutical industry; May and Baker Pharmaceuticals Ltd. invested £2M in new production facilities for Samorin.

For the studies at Mkwaja Ranch, Tanzania, and at Muhaka Village, Coast Province, Kenya, the School in partnership with May and Baker Pharmaceuticals Ltd (James McAinsh), ILCA, ILRAD and the Ministry of Agriculture and Livestock Development of Kenya were given a Meritorious Award in the Technology Transfer Section of the Industry Year Award in 1986 for the successful implementation of Animal Health Packages for parasitic diseases in developing countries.

However, the long term consequences are uncertain in that no new drugs for ruminants have appeared on the market, largely because trypanocides are not seen as a profitable product by the pharmaceutical industry. At the same time, drug resistance is an ever increasing problem.

2012
The first students graduate from the BSc programme in Veterinary Biosciences.

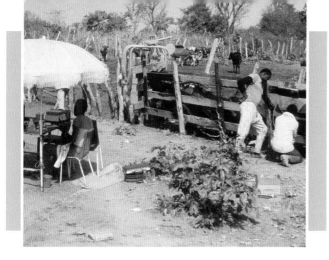

Dennis Hagan OBE, BVMS 1959

'I worked with a team to keep the truly veterinary charity VETAID active and financially sustainable. During this time I visited many worthwhile projects in Kenya, Mozambique and Somalia. Memories of aged grandparents wonderfully supporting and educating large families of grandchildren, where a generation of parents had succumbed to disease.

Observing remote village women learning to look after and multiply stock, then again watching very happy village children playing football with a blown up contraceptive using binder twine as an outer skin. Yes, a deeply humbling yet stimulating lesson in many ways'.

Investigations in the field

The Use of Genetic Resistance

Trypanotolerant breeds, mainly N'Dama, are a major option for sustainable livestock development in tsetse-infested countries of West and Central Africa. Resistance traits have also been identified in East Africa in certain *Bos indicus* types and are being exploited.

West and Central Africa

With scientists from Glasgow, the ITC, ILRAD and ILCA a continental programme evolved on the genetic resistance of breeds of livestock to trypanosomiasis, a trait referred to as trypanotolerance. The outcome of research over two decades was of major significance, identifying a significant alternative/addition for disease control in tsetse-infested Africa. The research focussed on the most widespread trypanotolerant breed of cattle, the N'Dama.

The main questions to be addressed were was the N'Dama truly resistant to the trypanosomiasis and if so did the resistance have a genetic basis or was it acquired and was the N'Dama, which was physically smaller then the main European breeds, less productive, as was widely believed?

It was shown that trypanotolerance is a powerful genetic trait characterised by the ability to resist anaemia and control parasitaemia. Both traits are repeatable, genetically controlled and heritable, and positively correlated to productivity, as computed using all major production traits. Furthermore, resistance can be enhanced by previous exposure and by dietary supplementation.

The N'Dama is as productive as other breeds in areas of zero or low tsetse risk, while in areas of higher risk it is the only breed that can survive without drugs. Other attributes, based on field observations were that N'Dama and West African Shorthorn appeared to possess traits almost akin to wildlife that allow them to survive and be productive in humid and subhumid regions. These include resistance to other endemic diseases such as tick-borne diseases, dermatophilosis (a massive problem) and helminthiasis. There is also evidence of greater heat tolerance, water conservation and ability to scavenge. Trypanotolerant breeds, mainly N'Dama, are a major option for sustainable livestock development in tsetse-infested areas of West and Central Africa.

East Africa

There have been several reports from East Africa of reduced susceptibility to trypanosomiasis in various types of *Bos indicus* cattle as well as indigenous sheep and goats.

In the 1960s, Matt Cunningham pointed out that thousands of local East African Zebu cattle around the shores of Lake Victoria survived despite continuous tsetse challenge. Then at Kilifi Plantations, 2/3 Sahiwal-1/3 Ayrshire were found to be more resistant than 1/3 Sahiwal-2/3 Ayrshire to trypanosomiasis, as judged by requirement of fewer treatments. This was of economic benefit to the rancher, as both cattle types were equally productive.

Several studies carried out in the 1990s by Glasgow in collaboration with Kenya Trypanosomiasis Research Institute also showed marked differences in susceptibility in *Bos indicus* types such as the Orma Boran which exhibited significant resistance to the disease. At the same time, imported *Bos taurus* breeds such as Ayrshire/Friesian have proved disastrously susceptible.

Glasgow played a catalytic role in highlighting the importance of trypanotolerance as a major strategy for the control of African trypanosomiasis in domestic livestock. Thus in some tsetse-infested regions trypanotolerant breeds can be productive where other breeds succumb, while in other breeds, differences in susceptibility can be profitable because of fewer requirements for treatment.

It could be said that Glasgow helped fulfil a vision of Lord Delamere in Kenya over a century ago in 1907: that it should be possible to breed animals 'immune to every known disease….. that would even penetrate tsetse areas.'

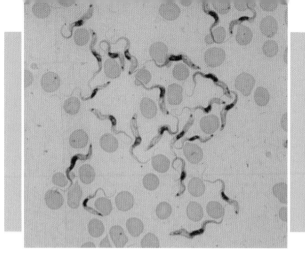

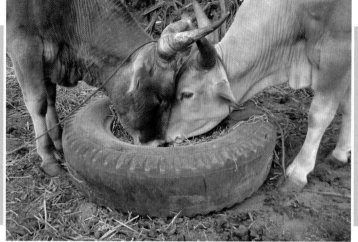

Human African trypanosomiasis (Sleeping Sickness)

Another very significant contribution from Glasgow has been in the field of Human African Trypanosomiasis (HAT), also known as sleeping sickness. The disease poses a serious threat to millions of Africans and the available treatments carry major risks. At present all patients die if not treated, while current treatment with intravenous melarsoprol leads to a severe post-treatment reactive encephalopathy in 10 percent of patients, half of whom die giving an overall fatality rate from the drug of 5 percent. The lack of a suitable animal model of the disease in humans has been a serious handicap. However, in research led by Frank Jennings followed by extensive neuropathogenetic work over the last twenty years by Peter Kennedy and Jean Rodgers, major achievements have been made. A mouse model employing *Trypansoma brucei brucei* developed by Frank Jennings in 1979 is now recognised worldwide as the gold standard, mimicking the neuropathology of the brain disease in HAT patients dying from the disease. Its use has led both to the understanding of key underlying mechanisms of the brain damage and the identification of new therapeutic targets for innovative drug therapy.

The mouse model of sleeping sickness was also used to identify new approaches to treatment, including combination chemotherapy. In a breakthrough of massive potential, Peter Kennedy and his research team have recently produced and tested in the mouse model a drug called complexed melarsoprol that can be given orally, is non-toxic and curative. Plans are now under way for carrying out a Phase IIa study of complexed melarsoprol in patients with CNS stage *T.b. rhodesiense* HAT in Uganda. If successful, this would be a breakthrough as there has never been a safe, orally available effective drug for HAT.

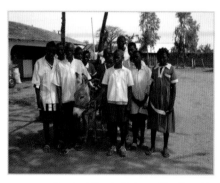

Sambel Kundu School. The Gambia

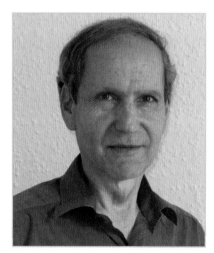

Peter Kennedy

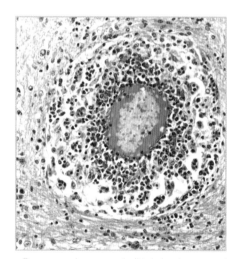

Severe meningoencephalitis in bovine caused by Trypanosoma brucei brucei

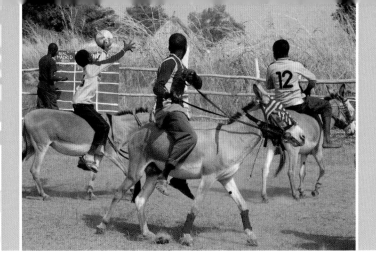

Donkey ball in The Gambia

Return to The Gambia

Recently David Sutton and Patrick Pollock of the Weipers Centre for Equine Welfare have been working in conjunction with the Gambia Horse and Donkey Trust (GHDT) to investigate a devastating outbreak of an unknown neurological disease which has caused a high mortality rate in the working horses and donkeys of the region. This emerging disease has in turn had profound effects on the local economy, and both animal and human welfare.

Work by a large group of scientists at both Glasgow and Liverpool Universities has now shown that a neurological disease is developing after infection with a trypanosome in the *T. brucei/evansi/equiperdum* group. The most recent piece in this puzzle has been the positive identification, using immunohistochemistry, of *Trypanosoma sp.* organisms in the brain of affected individuals.

The GHDT is a registered charity founded by Stella Marsden and her sister Heather Armstrong to alleviate rural poverty by increasing the productivity of working horses and donkeys though animal welfare and management education. Their vision was to help people to help themselves. Given the small size of the charity it has been tremendously productive and effective at improving the welfare of both the working equidae and the local community around its headquarters at Sambel Kunda.

Many undergraduate and postgraduate vets from Glasgow Veterinary School have volunteered and visited this unique clinic in West Africa, helping not only with animal care but with teaching in the school, and building a library and a skills' centre for women.

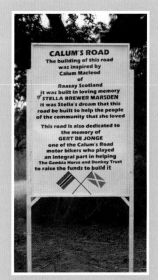

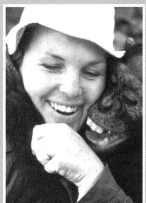

Stella Marsden

Calum's Road

Another development to which Glasgow contributed was the construction of a 7.5km road from the village to the river trading post, crossing swampland. Prior to construction of this road several local people had drowned during the wet season when attempting to reach the river crossing. Before her death in 2008, Stella Marsden had proposed to rebuild this road above swamp level, to allow safe passage throughout the year. This was inspired by crofter Calum Macleod of Raasay, who single-handedly connected his croft to the main road on the island of Raasay, as told in 'Calum's Road' written by Roger Hutchinson.

Heather Armstrong together with the villagers, and significant funding from the Highland Bikers, undertook the mammoth task, of rebuilding the road. After a number of local speeches, and as recorded on Gambian radio, David Sutton kicked off on his fiddle with the strathspey 'Calum's Road' before Patrick Pollock and his pipes led a colourful procession along the new road.

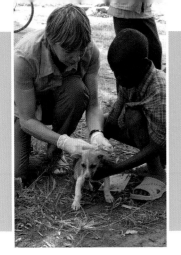
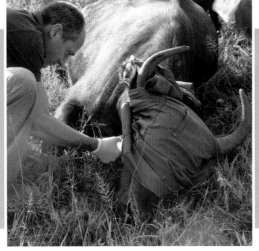
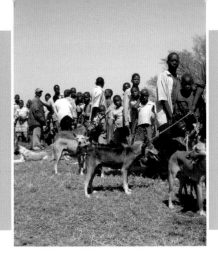

Control of other enzootic, epizootic and zoonotic diseases

Sarah Cleaveland, current Professor of Comparative Epidemiology in the Institute of Biodiversity Animal Health and Comparative Medicine and Associate Academic in the School of Veterinary Medicine, is leading several projects in East Africa on viral diseases of animals. She and her team are studying foot and mouth disease in wildlife and livestock in Tanzania as well as carrying out a vaccination trial against malignant catarrhal fever, a disease which has serious impact on livestock for pastoral communities. She is also an integral member of a team which plans to eliminate rabies in low income countries. According to the WHO, recent increases in human rabies deaths in South America and parts of Africa and Asia are evidence that the disease is re-emerging as a serious public health issue. The most cost-effective strategy for preventing rabies in people is by eliminating rabies in dogs through animal vaccinations. Funding has been obtained from the Bill and Melinda Gates Foundation which is being spent rolling out a canine vaccination programme – targeting domestic dogs – in three areas, Tanzania, Kwa Zulu Natal in South Africa and the Visayas archipelago of the Philippines.

Professor Cleaveland's team has also received additional support for epidemiological analysis of the data generated from the Gates/WHO project. This research is led by Glasgow Professor Dan Haydon, Director of the Institute of Biodiversity, Animal Health and Comparative Medicine. It is hoped that vaccination will eventually lead to the complete elimination of both dog and human rabies in these areas.[176]

Sarah Cleaveland has also been instrumental in developing multidisciplinary integrated human and animal health research programmes in East Africa. Following on from a project to investigate zoonotic diseases in urban and rural communities in Kenya, linked with the Centres for Disease Control and Prevention in Atlanta and the Kenya Medical Research Institute, she is now embarking on a project to investigate the epidemiology of three bacterial zoonoses, leptospirosis, brucellosis and Q-fever, in northern Tanzania, funded by the US National Institutes of Health and the UK BBSRC. This project is building on results of a human febrile surveillance study, carried out by scientists from the Kilimanjaro Christian Medical Center and Duke University, which shows that these zoonotic pathogens are the cause of disease in a high proportion (>20 percent) of people admitted to hospital with febrile illness.

This current project brings together human and animal health researchers with social scientist Jo Sharp from Glasgow, to assess the burden of these zoonoses, identify the most important risk factors in different livestock-keeping communities, and to help design appropriate prevention and control strategies.

Sarah Cleaveland has recently been appointed as Visiting Professor of the Nelson Mandela Africa Institute for Science and Technology. This is a new institution established in northern Tanzania, which aims to develop world-class international research that addresses the development goals of Africa.

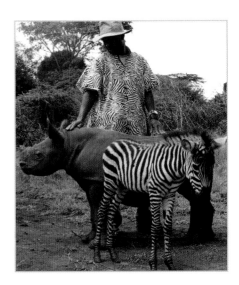

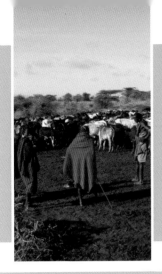

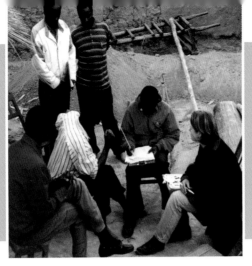

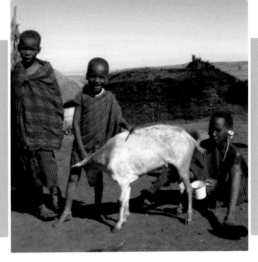

Primary health care technology transfer: bovine mastitis

Julie Fitzpatrick, then Professor of Farm Animal Medicine continued the Glasgow tradition, developing a project to alleviate poverty and improve animal health and welfare by implementing disease control programmes in the emerging smallholder dairy sector in Tanzania.

The project, funded by the DFID informed farmers how to recognise and treat mastitis, a condition which many involved in looking after dairy cows noticed, but which they did not specifically recognise as a disease, resulting in low treatment and cure rates. The project was deemed a huge success by local communities in Tanga, in the northern coastal region and in Iringa, the cooler hilly southern region of the country. The compliance rate of participating farms was 100 percent, mostly due to the excellent communication skills of the PhD students involved, both British and Tanzanian, but also due to the very attractive certificates provided to farmers on the completion of the work! The research team were delighted to see the certificates proudly displayed on the walls of rural villages over many subsequent years.

During travels around Tanzania, including to Sokoine University of Agriculture in Morogoro, Julie Fitzpatrick met vets, farmers and university staff who remembered well the original 'Glasgow Vets' who had helped to establish veterinary training, especially ruminant clinical training, decades before. Many anecdotes were fondly told.

Reflections on the African diaspora: an everlasting bond

McIntyre, Weipers and Urquhart started the ball rolling and were supported and followed by many colleagues over the years. Initially, The Rockefeller Foundation was the major enabler, with memorable meetings always with several Glaswegians present. Over the last fifty years the Glasgow Veterinary School has been in most countries in Africa and has built up a unique partnership of mutual benefit. Major long term research programmes have been established to the benefit of both man and animals and the collaborative links continue to this day.

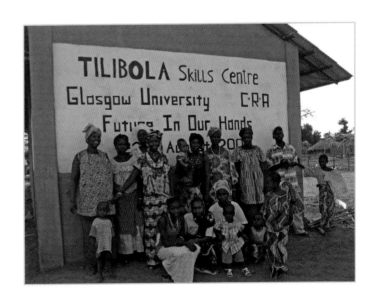

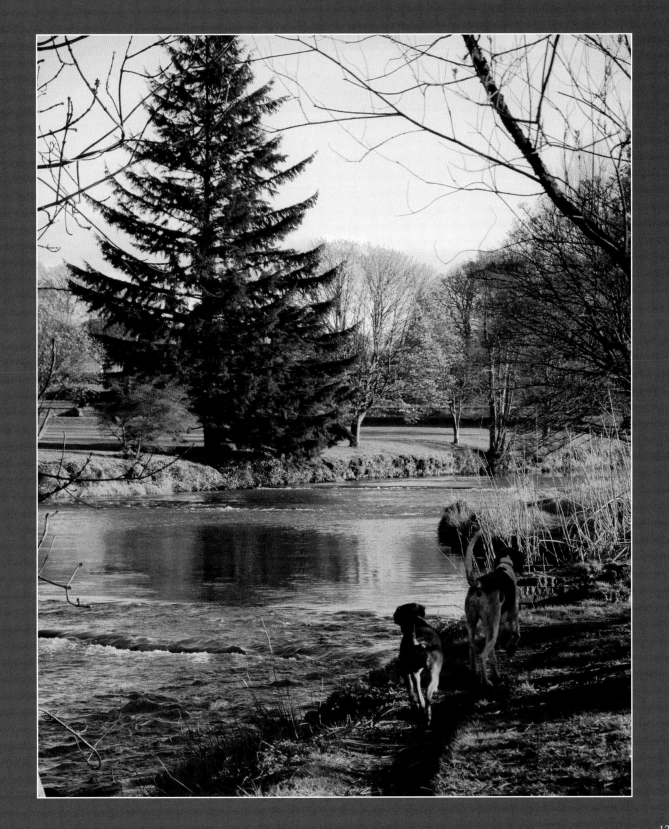

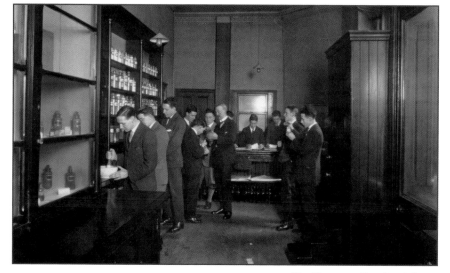

Afterword

The 150th anniversary has provided the stimulus
and opportunity to reflect on the School's history
from its humble beginnings in 1862. This book is
for our global alumni, our staff and students,
our profession as well as our donors and our
public supporters. In 2012, The University of
Glasgow Veterinary School has an outstanding
international reputation for its leading contributions
to veterinary medicine. Through its interdisciplinary
approach it has delivered world-leading advances in
veterinary education and research. What is the magic
essence of the School's success? Two remarkable
visionary and inspiring men were pivotal, James
McCall and William Weipers, both from Ayrshire.
McCall, our founder in 1862, who graduated from
The 'Dick' Veterinary School in Edinburgh saw the
opportunity to begin a veterinary school in Glasgow
in his late twenties. Through his strenuous efforts
over fifty years McCall raised the Glasgow Veterinary
College from humble beginnings to a School with
national status.

University of Glasgow

In 1949 William Weipers became Director of
Veterinary Education when the College was
integrated into the Faculty of Medicine at
The University.

This was a pivotal event in our history. Weipers had
a unique vision for the profession, namely, that it
should be closely aligned to human medicine in the
concept of 'One Medicine'. He created a centre of
international recognition and regard and a philosophy
that determined the future of the profession
throughout the world. Weipers complemented an
already gifted staff at the old College at Buccleuch
Street, by making a series of inspired appointments,
both veterinary surgeons and science graduates in
medicine, surgery, pathology, parasitology, virology,
physiology and biochemistry that produced a Nobel
Laureate, Fellows of the Royal Society and many
Fellows of the Royal Society of Edinburgh.

Weipers and his team led a well defined master
plan that evolved over the next sixty years,
whereby the new sciences and technologies were
embraced into the established disciplines in a well
defined infrastructure, with clear goals: classical
departments were encouraged to work in a range
of interdisciplinary teams for both teaching and
research; teaching was clinically driven, with
hands-on clinical and surgical training; national and
international interactions were essential; research
was based on the concept of one medicine, namely,
comparative medicine.

The *esprit de corps* was possibly the most
important component of the magic essence.
From the beginning in 1862, a Glasgow team spirit
progressively evolved during the Buccleuch Street
era. This *esprit de corps* was retained by Weipers
and his team during the integration of the old Vet
College into The University, despite rapid expansion.
Weipers and his senior lieutenants' genius was not
only to gather the best of staff, but also to generate
and sustain a pervading ambience of motivation,
entrepreneurship, blue-sky thinking, and interaction.
The management style ensured that all personnel
were recognised, appreciated and felt part of
'the team'.

The Pharmacy, Buccleuch Street

Weipers' vision for the School could only be realised by building new facilities on one site. The ideal location for this strategy was provided when The University obtained Garscube Estate in the West End of Glasgow. Moreover, Garscube was only 15 minutes from the main Campus, and from Cochno Farm Estate. The clinical facilities, the McCall Building, built in 1954, were followed by new buildings for the pre-and paraclinical departments in 1968, then by several smaller research facilities. In the 1990s and following major fund-raising campaigns an ambitious building programme was initiated. Over the next twenty years at the cost of multi-millions, new equine, farm animal and small animal facilities, and research laboratories, have been completed to take the School forward in the 21st Century.

While Glasgow is one of the world's great universities, the fourth oldest in the UK, from the beginning Weipers encouraged global interaction with the 'best' irrespective of location. In the early 1960s, Glasgow's attention turned towards Africa where most countries where gaining their independence but had very few qualified veterinary surgeons. Glasgow Veterinary School played a major role in the development of veterinary schools in East Africa and later in establishing major international and regional research centres. The African experience had a significant influence in Glasgow's own teaching and training approach and also our research interest in tropical diseases. Many Glasgow vet school staff and students have visited and worked in Africa over the last fifty years and continue to do so.

Glasgow Veterinary School has become a major world centre for virology, cancer and parasitology research, epidemiology and informatics, and technology transfer, making major advances in animal and human health. It provides a clinical service for animal across the UK from outstanding premises for both companion and farm animals. The Glasgow approach to teaching revolutionised veterinary education in the UK and became the blue print for many veterinary schools worldwide.

Glasgow's greatest achievement and contribution to the veterinary profession has been our progeny. At one time job advertisements in the Veterinary Record stated 'only Glasgow Graduates need apply'. Weipers identified world class staff. These stars spawned heirs. The consequence was innumerable eminent academics and world class researchers, often one and the same, Heads and Principals of veterinary schools throughout the world, Directors of research institutes, leaders of commerce, successful entrepreneurs, senior members of international organisations, Knights of the Realm, a President of a Country, famous authors and highly regarded general practitioners.

What more can be said other than the last 150 years have been an amazingly successful journey.

New and exciting challenges are now facing Glasgow and the profession in teaching, research and commercialisation. There are the questions of specialisation and speciation posing the dilemma of the omnicompetent veterinary surgeon.

The revolution in molecular biology and information technology has led to increasing collaboration and a common research approach across the biomedical sciences in Glasgow. To facilitate this interaction, in 2010 the new Principal, Anton Muscatelli, put in place a major structural reorganisation of the University which brought together the research activities across the Faculties into new research Institutes whilst the teaching responsibilities remained within the Schools of Medicine, Veterinary Medicine and Biomedical and Life Sciences. This matrix which epitomizes the concept of 'One Medicine' sits within a single new College. The new structure is providing exciting new opportunities for research, and cross disciplinary collaboration exemplified by the ever growing research income of Glasgow's veterinary scientists.

The School 'belongs to Glasgow'. Its history and ethos reflect those of the great city it is part of. Looking to the future the School reflects the City's motto 'Let Glasgow (continue to) Flourish'.

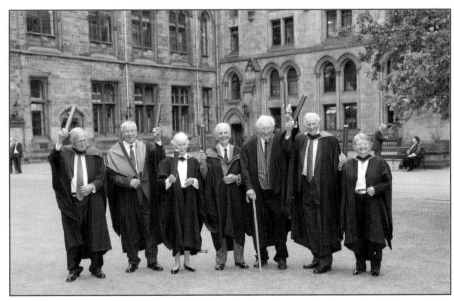

Former vet students from 1940s and 1950s finally graduate at the University of Glasgow 2010

Appendices

Heads of Glasgow Veterinary School 1862-2012

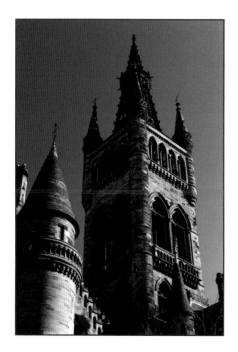

Principals of Glasgow Veterinary College	Dates
Professor James McCall	1862-1915
Mr Hugh Begg	1915-1917
Professor Sydney Gaiger	1917-1922
Dr Arthur Whitehouse	1922-1944
Mr Donald Campbell	1944-1945
Mr Albert Forsyth	1946-1949

Director of Veterinary Education	Dates
William Weipers	1949-1968

Deans of the Faculty of Veterinary Medicine	Dates
Sir William Weipers	1968-1974
Professor Ian McIntyre	1974-1977
Professor William Mulligan	1977-1980
Professor Donald Lawson	1980-1983
Professor Tom Douglas	1983-1986
Sir James Armour	1986-1991
Professor Norman Wright	1991-1999
Professor Andrea Nolan	1999-2004
Professor Stuart Reid	2005-2010

Heads of School of Veterinary Medicine	Dates
Professor Stuart Reid	2010-2011
Professor Ewan Cameron	2011-

Honorary Degrees and Fellowships

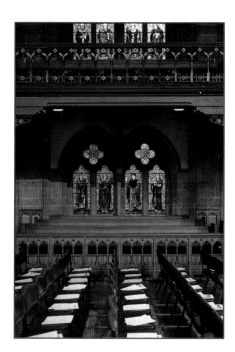

Honorary degrees (DVMS)

	Date awarded
Sir William Lee Weipers	1982
Mrs Elisabeth Svendsen	1992
Mr Alastair Robert Wilson Porter	1993
Dr Gordon James Piller	1997
Professor Roderick Campbell	1999
Mrs Daphne Marjorie Sheldrick	2000
Ms Annette Crosbie	2000
Dr Judith MacArthur Clark	2001
Ernest Jackson Lawson, Right Honourable, Lord Soulsby of Swaffham Prior	2001
Professor Feshea Gebreab	2001
Professor William Fleming Hoggan Jarrett	2002
Dr William Barr Martin	2002
Dr Gardner Murray	2003
Professor Neil Gorman	2004
Professor Craig Sharp	2005
Professor David Onions	2006
Mrs Stella Marsden	2006
Professor John Preston	2007
Mr Ian James Galloway	2009
Mrs Alison Bruce	2012

Honorary Fellowships

	Date awarded
Mr James Wight	1998
Mrs Alison Bruce	1998
Dr Valerie Cairns	1999
Mr James McAinsh	2000
Professor George Gettinby	2001
Mr George Barr	2002
Mr Harry Pfaff	2003
Mr Harry Wilson	2004

Staff List 2012

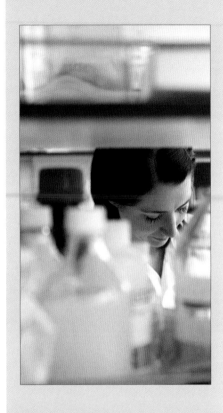

Research and Teaching

Allan, Dr Kathryn (Wellcome Training Fellow)
Anderson, Prof Jim (Professor of Veterinary Neurology and Neurosurgery)
Auckburally, Mr Adam (Senior Veterinary Clinician)
Barrett, Mrs Ute (Learning Technologist)
Bell, Mr Andrew (University Clinician)
Bell, Mr Rory (Senior Veterinary Clinician)
Bennett, Prof David (Professor of Small Animal Clinical Studies)
Brannan, Mrs Nicola (Diagnostic Imager)
Burnside, Miss Shona (Radiotherapist)
Calvo, Mr Ignacio (Lecturer/Clinician in Small Animal Orthopaedic Surgery)
Cameron, Prof Ewan (Head of School)
Cameron, Mrs Gillian (Diagnostic Imager)
Campbell, Miss Tracey (University Teacher)
Denwood, Dr Matthew (Lecturer in Production Animal Health (Large Animal Clinical Sciences and Public Health))
Dowell, Dr Fiona (Senior Lecturer)
Ellis, Dr Kathryn (Senior University Clinician)
Fishwick, Dr Graham (Lecturer)
Fitzpatrick, Prof Julie (Professor of Food Security)
Flaherty, Prof Derek (Senior University Vet Clinician)
Garcia Gonzalez, Miss Beatriz (Lecturer in Veterinary Pathology)
Geraghty, Mr Timothy (Lecturer)
Graham, Dr Libby (Veterinary Clinician)
Grant, Miss Melanie (Small Animal Physiotherapist)
Haining, Ms Hayley (Lecturer)
Haley, Dr Allison (University Clinician in Neurology)
Hammond, Mr Gawain (Senior University Clinician)
Hammond, Mrs Jennifer (University Teacher)
Hastie, Dr Peter (Research Fellow)
Helm, Miss Jenny (University Clinician in Small Animal Oncology)
Houston, Dr Fiona (Senior Research Fellow)
Hulme-Moir, Dr Lisa (Veterinary Clinician)
Jackson, Dr Mark (Senior Lecturer)
Jeffcoate, Dr Ian (Senior Lecturer)
Johnston, Dr Pamela (Senior Lecturer)
Jonsson, Prof Nicholas (Professor of Animal Production and Public Health)

King, Dr Alison (Senior Lecturer)
Knottenbelt, Prof Clare (Professor of Small Animal Medicine and Oncology)
Lamm, Dr Catherine (Lecturer in Veterinary Pathology)
Love, Prof Sandy (Professor of Equine Clinical Studies)
Maceachern, Dr Karen (University Teacher)
Marshall, Dr John (Lecturer in Equine Surgery)
Marshall, Mr William (University Clinician in Small Animal Orthopaedic Surgery)
McAllister, Mrs Angela (University Clinician)
McBrearty, Mrs Alix (Veterinary Clinician in Small Animal Oncology)
McLauchlan, Mr Gerard (University Veterinary Clinician in Small Animal Medicine)
McLaughlin, Dr Mark (Lecturer)
Mellor, Prof Dominic (Professor of Epidemiology and Veterinary Public Health)
Mihm Carmichael, Dr Monika (Senior Lecturer)
Morris, Dr Joanna (Senior Lecturer)
Nicolson, Dr Lesley (Senior Lecturer)
Parkin, Dr Tim (Senior Research Fellow)
Pawson, Dr Pat (Senior Veterinary Clinician)
Penderis, Prof Jacques (Professor of Comparative Neurology)
Pollock, Mr Patrick (Senior University Clinician)
Pratschke, Ms Kathryn (Senior University Clinician)
Ramsey, Prof Ian (Professor of Small Animal Medicine)
Reardon, Mr Richard (Research Assistant)
Roberts, Prof Mark (Professor of Molecular Bacteriology)
Steele, Mr Billy (Senior Lecturer)
Sullivan, Prof Martin (Professor of Veterinary Surgery and Diagnostic Imaging)
Sutton, Dr David (Senior University Veterinary Clinician)
Swiderski, Dr Michal (Associate Academic)
Voute, Dr Lance (Senior Veterinary Clinician)
Wessmann, Dr Annette (Senior University Clinician)
Wolfe, Miss Lissann (Teaching Assistant)
Yam, Dr Philippa (Senior Lecturer)

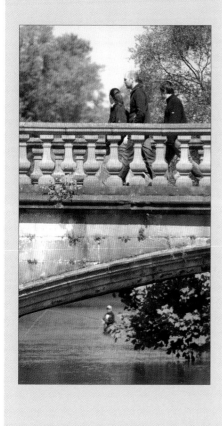

Associate Academics

Bain, Dr Maureen
Barry, Prof Dave
Beczkowski, Dr Pawel
Bellingham, Dr Michelle
Boden, Dr Lisa
Borland, Dr Gillian
Britton, Dr Collette
Caporale, Dr Marco
Cleaveland, Prof Sarah
Devaney, Prof Eileen
Dickens, Dr Nick
Donaldson, Dr Mary
Eckersall, Prof David
Edgar, Dr Julia
Elliott, Dr Elspeth
Evans, Prof Neil
Everest, Dr Paul
Gallagher, Dr Alice
Gillan, Dr Victoria
Hosie, Prof Margaret
Huser, Dr Camille
Jarrett, Prof Ruth
Kao, Prof Rowland
Kilbey, Dr Anna
Kinnaird, Dr Jane
Lake, Ms Annette
Logan, Miss Nicola
Loughrey, Dr Christopher
Maccallum, Dr Amanda
Mackay, Mrs Annie
Macleod, Dr Annette
Maitland, Ms Kirsty
Marchetti, Dr Barbara
Matthews, Dr Louise

Mckeegan, Dr Dorothy
Mcmonagle, Mrs Elizabeth
Montgomery, Mrs Dorothy
Morgan, Prof Iain
Morrison, Dr Liam
Murgia, Dr Claudio
Nasir, Prof Lubna
Nechyporuk-Zloy, Dr Volodymyr
Neil, Prof James
O'Hare, Dr Anthony
O'Shaughnessy, Prof Peter
Page, Prof Tony
Palmarini, Prof Massimo
Ratinier, Dr Maxime
Rich, Dr Tina
Roberts, Dr Brett
Robinson, Dr Jane
Rodgers, Dr Jean
Shaw, Dr Andrew
Sherry, Dr Aileen
Shiels, Prof Brian
Slater, Dr Nicholas
Smith, Prof David
Stear, Prof Michael
Terry, Mrs Anne
Weir, Dr Willie
Wilkes, Dr Jonathan
Willett, Prof Brian
Winter, Dr Alan

Management and Support

Ainsworth, Mrs Julie (Veterinary Nurse)
Allan, Ms Kirsty (Animal Care Assistant)
Allan, Ms Linda (Receptionist)
Allan, Miss Lisa (Veterinary Nurse (Out of Hours)
Anderson, Ms Lois (Specialist Veterinary Nurse)
Armstrong, Mrs Jennifer (Receptionist)
Barron, Mr Ronnie (Laboratory Manager)
Bell, Miss Karen (Veterinary Nurse)
Bell, Mrs Margaret (Technician)
Best, Mrs Anne (Administrative Assistant)
Bowie, Mrs Andrea (Technician)
Boyce, Miss Emma (Specialist Veterinary Nurse)
Burbidge, Miss Cecily (Equine Veterinary Nurse)
Calvo, Ms Gillian (Specialist Practitioner Vet Nurse)
Carmody, Miss Grace (Administrative Assistant)
Carver, Miss Donna (Specialist Veterinary Nurse)
Chestnut, Ms Carol (Stockperson)
Chiodetto, Ms Sarah (Head of Adminstration)
Chirwa, Mrs Lumba (Administrative Assistant)
Constable, Mrs Pauline (Secretary/Receptionist)
Cordner, Mr Ian (Stockperson)
Crozier, Mr Stephen (Stockperson)
Daly, Mrs Leigh (Veterinary Nurse)
Darby, Mrs Lynn (Senior Veterinary Nurse)
Davis, Miss Adelle (Animal Care Assistant)
Denman, Mrs Fiona (Administrative Assistant)
Drummond, Miss Holly (Equine Groom)
Drummond, Mr Kenneth (Stockperson)
Dunbar, Mrs Dawn (Technician)
Elder, Mrs Claire (Clerical Assistant)
Fallon, Mrs Linda (Administrative Assistant)
Ferry, Miss Leighann (Veterinary Nurse)
Fitzpatrick, Miss Janice (Technical Assistant)
Flanagan, Mrs Claire (Administrative Assistant)
Fontaine, Ms Sam (Specialist Practitioner
Veterinary Nurse)
Fraser, Mrs Maria (Administrative Assistant)
French, Dr Anne (Senior University Clinician)
Fuentes, Mr Manuel (Technician)
Gatherer, Miss Mary (Head Equine Nurse)
Gault, Mr Robert (Head Stockperson)
George, Ms Linda (Equine Veterinary Nurse)
Gilchrist, Mr Fraser (Finance Assistant)

Gordon, Miss Elizabeth (Receptionist)
Graham, Miss Gail (Administrative Assistant)
Graham, Ms Jane (Finance Manager)
Haggarty, Ms Jennifer (Administrative Assistant)
Hamilton, Mrs Janis (Senior Nursing Tutor)
Harvie, Mr James (Technician)
Hunter, Miss Gail (Senior Veterinary Nurse)
Hutchinson, Mrs Caroline (Operations Manager)
Ironside, Miss Gillian (Clerical Assistant)
Irvine, Mr Richard (Technician)
Jackson, Ms Lorraine (Specialist Veterinary Nurse)
Kelly, Miss Sarah (Veterinary Nurse (night))
Kerr, Mrs Jill (Administrative Assistant)
Lawless, Mrs Nan (Administrative Assistant)
Macdonald, Miss Sharon (Veterinary Nurse)
MacKay, Ms Patricia (Receptionist)
Macleod, Miss Moira (Veterinary Nurse)
Macmillan, Mr Iain (Laboratory Manager)
Macrae, Miss Arlene (Undergraduate School
Manager)
Marshall, Mrs Cheryl (Administrative Assistant)
Marshall, Mrs Leigh (Technician)
Mccoll, Mr Malcolm (Stockperson)
Mccoll, Miss Stacey (Veterinary Nurse)
Mccomb, Mrs Pamela (Head Veterinary Nurse)
Mcdonald, Miss Lyn (Veterinary Nurse)
Mcdonald, Mr Mike (Laboratory Manager)
Mcelhill, Miss Catriona (General Support Nurse)
Mcgoldrick, Mr James (Technician)
Mcgrane, Mrs Janet (Administrative Assistant)
Mcguigan, Mr Michael (Technician)
Mcindoe, Ms Caroline (Veterinary Nurse)
Mckendrick, Miss Lynn (Animal Care Assistant)
Mckenna, Mrs Iris (Receptionist)
Mcnaught, Mr Iain (Technician)
Mercer, Mr Alistair (Groom/Stockperson)
Munro, Miss Shona (Veterinary Nurse)
Murdoch, Miss Annette (Laundry Assistant)
Murphy, Mr Steven (Veterinary Nurse)
Murray, Miss Janice (Veterinary Nurse)
Neil, Ms Laura (Small Animal Hospital
Administrator)
Newham, Mr David (Technician)
Norden, Mrs Julie (Administrative Assistant)
O'Neil, Mr Brian (Human Resources Manager)
Oxford, Ms Lynn (Technician)

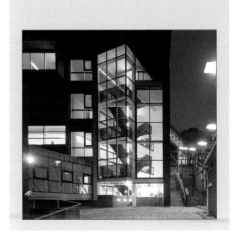

Paterson, Miss Rachael (Insurance Clerk)
Purvis, Mr Alan (Technician)
Raju, Mrs Pritpal (Finance Assistant)
Ralston, Mrs Elspeth (Groom)
Ram, Mrs Laura (Administrative Assistant)
Reid, Mr Kyle (Animal Care Assistant)
Reid, Mr Paul (Animal Care Assistant)
Rennie, Mrs Sharmila (Technician)
Reynolds, Miss Kathleen (Technician)
Richardson, Miss Lorna (Veterinary Nurse)
Scott, Mrs Clarice (Administrative Assistant)
Sharp, Miss Paula (Commercial Director)
Smith, Miss Jessica (Veterinary Nurse)
Smith, Mrs Sharon (Senior Veterinary Nurse)
Stevenson, Mrs Marion (Technician)
Stewart, Ms Lindsay (Veterinary Nurse)
Storie, Miss Hannah (Groom)
Sullivan, Mrs Alison (Veterinary Nurse)
Tweedie, Miss Hilary (Special Veterinary Nurse)
Veselovska, Miss Lenka (Administrative Assistant)
Wall, Miss Jennifer (Veterinary Nurse)
Wallace, Ms Angela (Special Veterinary Nurse)
Wallace, Mrs Morag (Administrator)
Wason, Mrs Joyce (Manager)
Weir, Miss Fiona (Laboratory Assistant)
Whiteside, Miss Linda (Animal Care Assistant)
Wild, Mrs Jane (Administrative Assistant)
Williamson, Mr Kenny (Technician)
Wilson, Mrs Katie (Groom)
Wilson, Miss Patricia (Laboratory Worker)
Young, Miss Jordan (Equine Groom)

Emeritus, Honorary and Visiting Appointees

Professors Emeritus

Armour, Sir James
Duncan, Professor James
Holmes, Professor Peter
Lawson, Professor Donald
Mulligan, Professor William
Wright, Professor Norman

Professors Emeritus and Honorary Senior Research Fellows

Campo, Professor Saveria
Boyd, Professor Jack
Jarrett, Professor Oswald
Logue, Professor David
Murray, Professor Max
Parkins, Professor James
Tait, Professor Andrew
Taylor, Professor David
Reid, Professor Jacqueline
Solomon, Professor Sally

Honorary Senior Research Fellows

Addie, Dr Diane
Aughey, Mrs Elizabeth
Beeley, Dr Josie
Harvey, Dr Michael

Honorary Professors

Coia, Professor John
Doerig, Professor Christian
Ellis, Professor Shirley
Forbes, Professor Andrew
Knox, Professor David
Gorman, Professor Neil
Greet, Professor Timothy
Marr, Professor Celia
Mertens, Professor Peter
Onions, Professor David
Preston, Professor John
Trees, Sir Alexander

Visiting Professors

Argyle, Professor David
Bonagura, Professor John
Donachie, Professor William
Done, Professor Stan
Gilleard, Professor John
Gunn, Professor George
Hodgson, Professor David
Kambarage, Professor Dominic
Katunguka-Rwakishaya, Professor Eli
Knight, Professor Chris
Mcewan, Professor Scott
Mckellar, Professor Quintin
Morrison, Professor Ivan
Ndung'u, Professor Joseph
Reid, Professor Stuart
Reilly, Professor William

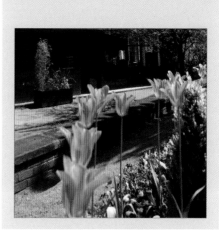

Honorary Appointees

Blyth, Dr Karen
Brown, Dr D
Fisher, Miss Donna
Forsythe, Mr Peter
Gettinby, Professor George
Gibbs, Dr Alison
Girling, Mr Simon
Harwood, Mr David
Hutchison, Mrs Pippa
Jackson, Dr Hilary
Johnston, Mr Norman
Lawrie, Mr Alistair
Lindley, Ms Samantha
Macleod, Mr Alistair
Matthews, Mr Andrew
Megahy, Mr Ian
Noddings, Ms Anne
Peplinski, Mr George
Purton, Dr Michael
Shearer, Mr Alan
Walker, Ms Sheena
Wotton, Dr Paul

Memorial Lectures

For the School's friends and supporters, alumni, members of the veterinary profession and civic society, the Weipers lectures, and more recently the McCall lectures are an important annual/biennial event. Over the past twenty years, there have been some outstanding speakers, many evoking strong memories of the Vet School.

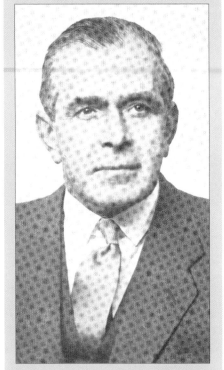

Sir William Weipers

Sir William Weipers Memorial Lectures

2011
'Husbandry regained: futures for animals in agriculture'
Professor John Webster, MA VetMB PhD MRCVS
Emeritus Professor of Animal Husbandry, University of Bristol

2009
'Stem cells and brain repair; hope or hype'
Professor Ian D Duncan, BVMS, PhD
Professor, Department of Medical Sciences, University of Wisconsin-Madison

2007
'Scotland and the Blue Revolution'
Professor Ronald J Roberts, CCT, BVMS, PhD, FRCPath, CBiol, FIBiol, FRSE, FRCVS
Institute of Aquaculture, University of Stirling

2005
'Sex and Exercise: Common Pathways, Different Outcomes'
Professor Lance Lanyon, CBE, BVSc, PhD, DSc, FMedSci, MRCVS
Principal, Royal Veterinary College, London

2003
'Pestilence and Public Health: The Continuing Threat'
Professor Sir John Arbuthnott, PhD, ScD, FRCPath, FRSE
Chairman of Greater Glasgow NHS Board

2001
'The Other Side of the Fence: A Glasgow Botanist and Whitehall'
Sir William Stewart, FRS, FRSE, President of the Royal Society of Edinburgh

1998
'Immunology: hitting back at bugs'
Professor Ian McConnell, FRSE, University of Cambridge

1996
'Mathematics and Medicine: A New Romance for the Next Millennium'
Professor George Gettinby, BSc, DPhil
Department of Statistics and Modelling Science, University of Strathclyde

1994
'Dr Finlay Meets Mr. Herriot'
Dr Kenneth C Calman, MD, PhD, FRCS (GlasEd), FRCP (LondEd.), FRCGP, FRCR, MFCM, FRSE, Chief Medical Officer, Department of Health, London

1991
'Out of Africa - Genetic Resistance: Nature's Contribution to a Global Problem'
Professor M Murray, BVMS, PhD, DVM, FRCPath, FRSE, MRCVS
Department of Veterinary Medicine, University of Glasgow

1990
'Veterinary Education: Horizons and Perspectives'
Dr A R Michell, BVetMed, BSc, PhD
Department of Veterinary Medicine, Royal Veterinary College, London

1989

'The Future and Relevance of Veterinary Research'
Professor F J Bourne, BVetMed, PhD
Director, AFRC Institute for Animal Health,
Compton

1988

'Cancer and AIDS: The Contribution
of Comparative Medicine'
Professor W F H Jarrett, FRS
Department of Veterinary Pathology,
University of Glasgow

1987

'The Grass on the Other Side'
Professor Ronald S Anderson, BVMS, PhD
Department of Animal Husbandry, University
of Liverpool

1986

'Behavioural Therapy: New Opportunities in
Canine and Feline Practice'
Professor Benjamin L Hart, DVM, PhD,
Department of Physiological Sciences, School of
Veterinary Medicine, University of California

1985

'The Price of Freedom'
Mr A R W Porter, CBE
Secretary and Registrar, The Royal College
of Veterinary Surgeons, London

1984

'The Scientific & Social Impacts of Recent
Advances in Biotechnology'
Sir William Henderson, FRS
Chairman, Horserace Betting Levy Board
Advisory Committee

1983

'A Common European Veterinary Policy'
Dr H J Bendixen, DrMed.Vet, Head Division
of Legislation relating to veterinary matters
and zootechnics, Commission of the European
Communities

1982

'Enhancement of the Human/Animal
Companion Bond'
Professor Leo K Bustad, BS, DVM, PhD
Dean, The College of Veterinary Medicine,
Washington State University

1981

'The Support of Veterinary Research'
The Lord Swann, FRS, Provost of Oriel College,
Oxford University

1980

'Science and the Seals: A Personal View'
Dr John Morton Boyd, FRSE, Director Scotland,
Nature Conservancy Council

1979

'Limits to Animal Production'
Sir Kenneth Blaxter, FRS, Director,
The Rowett Research Institute, Aberdeen

1978

'Limits to New Drug Research'
Sir James W Black, FRS
Director, Therapeutic Research, Wellcome Labs,
Beckenham

1977

'Reproduction in Wild Animals'
Professor R V Short, FRS, Director, MRC
Reproductive Biology Unit, Edinburgh

1976

'The International Veterinarian'
A G Beynon, CB, DVMS, President,
Royal College of Veterinary Surgeons

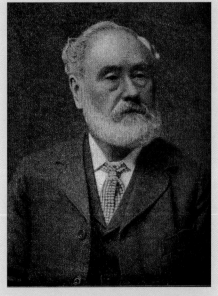

Professor James McCall

Professor James McCall Memorial Lectures

2012

'Plague; coming or going?'
Professor Stuart Reid, BVMS PhD DVM
DipECVPH FRSE MRCVS, Principal, Royal
Veterinary College

2010

'Human river blindness, cows and some
remarkable bacteria'
Professor Lord Trees BVM&S PhD DipEVPC
DVetMed(hc) MRCVS (Lord in 2012)

2008

'Viruses, vaccines, pandemics and paranoia'
Professor David Onions, DVMS

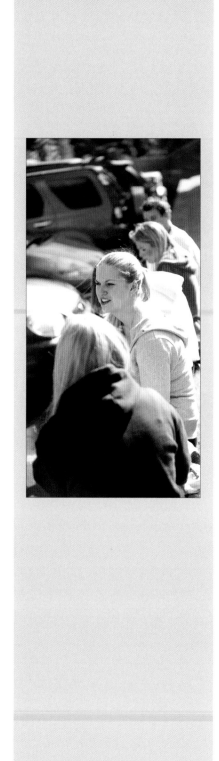

Photograph legends

School Executive 2012   Foreword
Front row: David Bennett,
Lubna Nasir, Caroline Hutchinson,
Ewan Cameron, Clare Knottenbelt,
Sarah Chiodetto
Back row: Sandy Love, Dom Mellor,
Nick Jonsson, Jim Anderson,
Jane Graham, Maureen Bain,
Paula Sharp

Professor James McCall   8

Sir William Weipers   28

Nursing staff 2010   43
Front Row: Janis Hamilton, Lynn Darby,
Sharon Smith, Jennifer Freytag,
Cheryl Mackie, Lynn McKendrick,
Lindsay Stewart
Back Row: Samantha Fontaine,
Kerry Melville,
Janice Murray

Bill Jarrett   52

Neurology Service 2012   74
Front row: Gillian Calvo,
Rodrigo Gutierrez
Back row: Annette Wessmann,
Jaques Penderis,
Jim Anderson, Maria Ortega

Orthopaedic Service 2010   76
David Bennett, William Marshall,
Ignacio Calvo, Russell Yeadon,
Damian Chase

Reproductive Physiology group 2012   80
Front Row: Dr Ana Monteiro.
Back Row: Jane Robinson,
Professor Peter O'Shaughnessy,
Janette Bonnar, Ian Jeffcoate,
Nicky Craig, Neil Evans,
Monika Mihm Carmichael,
Lynne Fleming.

Companion Animal Diagnostics,   87
Infectious Diseases Group
Front row: Dawn Dunbar,
Libby Graham, Kathleen Reynolds,
Andrea Bowie.
Back row: James McGoldrick,
Manuel Fuentes, Mike McDonald,
Leigh Marshall

Glasgow Veterinary School   90

Farm animal staff 2010:   94
Front Row: Thomas Wittek, Laura Beasley,
Kathryn Ellis, Isabelle Truyers
Back row: David Barrett, Lorenzo Viora,
David Logue, Diether Prins

Equine Staff 2012   97
David Sutton, Mary Gatherer,
Alexandra Raftery, Sandy love,
Elspeth Ralston, Linda George,
Cecily Burbidge, Jennifer Haggarty,
Padraig Kelly, Michael Cathcart,
Sylvia Maliye, John Marshall,
Jordan Young, Patrick Pollock
(and the horse is called Harley)

Oncology Service   99
Front Row: Jo Morris,
Clare Knottenbelt
Back Row: Matt Atherton,
Jenny Helm, Sam Fontaine

Conversion course, Kabete 1964   112

River Kelvin, Garscube Campus   126

Abbreviations

AFRC   Agricultural and Food Research Council
AGP   Alpha-1 Acid Glycoprotein
AIDS   Acquired immunodeficiency syndrome
ARC   Agricultural Research Council
APP   Acute Phase Proteins
AVMA   American Veterinary Medical Association
BBSRC   Biotechnology and Biological Sciences Research Council
BEVA   British Equine Veterinary Association
BoHV-2   Bovine Herpes Virus type 2
BPV   Bovine Papillomavirus
BVA   British Veterinary Association
BVMS   Bachelor of Veterinary Medicine and Surgery
CAL   Computer-Assisted Learning
CAV   Canine Adenovirus
CDV   Canine Distemper Virus
CBE   Commander of the British Empire
CGIAR   Consultative Group on International Agricultural Research
CHV   Canine Herpes Virus
CIDRU   Canine Infectious Diseases Unit
CLIVE   Computer-aided Learning In Veterinary Education
CPD   Continuing Professional Development
CPE   European Centre for the Clinical Proficiency Examination
CPIV   Canine Parainfluenza Virus
CPV   Canine Parvovirus
CSP   Clinical Scholars Programme
CT   Computed Tomography
CVR   Centre for Virus Research
DAO   Development and Alumni Office
DEFRA   Department for Environment, Food and Rural Affairs
DFID   Department for International Development
DNA   Deoxyribonucleic acid
DOA   Department of Agriculture
DVM   Diploma in Veterinary Medicine
EATRO   East African Trypanosomiasis Research Organisation
EAVE   European Association of Establishments for Veterinary Education

EAVRO   East African Veterinary Research Organisation
EBV   Epstein-Barr Virus
EC   European Commission
ECBHM   European College of Bovine Health Management
ECFVG   Educational Commission for Foreign Veterinary Graduates
ECVPH   European College of Veterinary Public Health
EM   Electron Microscopy
EMG   Electromyography
EMS   Extramural Studies
ERDF   European Regional Development Fund
ESR Plus   Erythrocyte Sedimentation Rate
EU   European Union
FAO   Food and Agriculture Organisation
FCoV   Feline Coronavirus
FeLV   Feline Leukaemia Virus
FIP   Feline Infectious Peritonitis
FIV   Feline Immunodeficiency Virus
FMD   Foot and Mouth Disease
FRCVS   Fellow of Royal College of Veterinary Surgeons
FSA   Food Standards Agency
FVU   Feline Virus Unit
GCPS   Glasgow Composite Pain Scale
GCPS- SF   Glasgow Composite Pain Scale Shortened Form
GHDT   Gambia Horse and Donkey Trust
GLASS   Garscube Learning and Social Space
GUVMA   Glasgow University Veterinary Medical Association
HAT   Human African Trypanosomiasis
HIV   Human Immunodeficiency Virus
HLA   Human Leukocyte Antigen
HTLV   Human T-cell Leukaemia Virus
IBAR   Interafrican Bureau of Animal Resources)
IBR   Infectious bovine rhinotracheitis
Ig   Immunoglobulin
ILCA   International Livestock Centre for Africa
ILRAD   International Laboratory for Research on Animal Diseases
ILRI   International Livestock Research Institute
ITC   International Trypanotolerance Centre
JSRV   Jaagsiekte Sheep Retrovirus
LRF   Leukaemia Research Fund
M.Sci   Master of Science

MA   Master of Arts
MC   Military Cross
MCF   Malignant Catarrhal Fever
Mg/Al/Cu   Magnesium/Aluminium/Copper
MHC   Major histocompatability complex
MHS   Meat Hygiene Service
MOODLE   Modular Object-Oriented Dynamic Learning Environment
MoU   Memorandum of Understanding
MP   Member of Parliament
MRC   Medical Research Council
MRCVS   Member of Royal College of Veterinary Surgeons
MRI   Magnetic Resonance Imaging
MVO   Member of the Victorian Order
NMVA   National Medical Veterinary Association
OAU   Organisation of African Unity
OBE   Order of the British Empire
ODA   Overseas Development Administration
OPA   Ovine Pulmonary Adenocarcinoma
OSCE   Objective Structured Clinical Examination
PCV   Packed Cell Volume
PDSA   People's Dispensary for Sick Animals
PhD   Doctor of Philosophy
PM   Post mortem
RAE   Researxh Assessment Exercise
RCVS   Royal College of Veterinary Surgeons
RDA   Riding for the Disabled
RNA   Ribonucleic acid
SAC   Scottish Agricultural College
SAH   Small Animal Hospital
SAVMA   Student American Veterinary Medical Association
SCPAHFS   Scottish Centre for Production Animal Health and Food Safety
SMART award   Small Funding Merit Award for Research and Technology
SSPCA   Scottish Society for the Prevention of Cruelty to Animals
TLTP   Teaching and Learning Technology Programme
UGC   University Grants Committee
VIE   Veterinary Informatics and Epidemiology
WHO   World Health Organisation
WUMP   Wellcome Unit of Molecular Parasitology

References

1. Glasgow Veterinary School 1862-1962 (1962) p4
2. The Royal College of Veterinary Surgeons 1844-1944 Centenary Commemoration Number, The Veterinary Record Vol 57 No 51 (1945) pp 599-677 p632
3. Carter, V, ed, Cotchin, E, The Royal Veterinary College London A Bicentenary History, Buckingham (1990) p13
4. Adair, W, The Glasgow Veterinary College (incorporated) Records of Eighty Years Progress (1941) p9
5. Obituary of James McCall in the Scottish Farmer 10th November (1915), University of Glasgow Archives DC 144/7/1
6. Weipers, WL, The Development of Veterinary Education in the West of Scotland. British Veterinary Journal (1975), 131, 3, pp3-16 p7
7. Adair, W, The Glasgow Veterinary College (incorporated) Records of Eighty Years Progress (1941) p9
8. Records of Anderson's Institution/Anderson's University/ Anderson's College www.strath.ac.uk/archives/ourcollections/xml/ institutionalarchives/recordsofandersonsinstitutionandersonsuniversity andersonscollege/(August 2011)
9. Moss, M, Rankin, M, Richmond L, Who, Where and When: The History & Constitution of the University of Glasgow (2001) p12
10. Anderson's College www.universitystory.gla.ac.uk/building/?id=35 (August 2011)
11. Adair, W, The Glasgow Veterinary College (incorporated) Records of Eighty Years Progress (1941) p9
12. Weipers, WL, The Development of Veterinary Education in the West of Scotland. British Veterinary Journal (1975), 131, 3, pp3-16 p8
13. Weipers, WL, The Development of Veterinary Education in the West of Scotland. British Veterinary Journal (1975), 131, 3, pp3-16 p5
14. Adair, W, The Glasgow Veterinary College (incorporated) Records of Eighty Years Progress (1941) p9
15. Glasgow Veterinary School 1862-1962 (1962) p5
16. Adair, W, The Glasgow Veterinary College (incorporated) Records of Eighty Years Progress (1941) p10
17. Armitage, G, The Thermometer as an Aid to Diagnosis in Veterinary Medicine, AP Muddiman, (1869)
18. Moss P, Moss M, Early History. Newsletter of the University of Glasgow Veterinary Faculty Issue No 6, November 1997, p3
19. Glasgow Veterinary College 1861-1874, University of Glasgow Archives Collection DC 144/7/6/1
20. Glasgow Veterinary School 1862-1962 (1962) p6
21. Scotland in the 19th Century. Index of statutes http://gdl.cdlr.strath.ac.uk/haynin/hayninindexstatute.html (August 2011)
22. Glasgow Veterinary School 1862-1962 (1962) p6
23. Blairtummock House Http://www.blairtummockhouse.org.uk/ (September 2011)
24. Obituary of James McCall in the Scottish Farmer 10th November 1915), University of Glasgow Archives Collection DC 144/7/1
25. Personal papers of Geraldine McCall
26. Weipers, WL, The Development of Veterinary Education in the West of Scotland. British Veterinary Journal (1975), 131, 3, pp3-16 p8
27. Macaulay, JW, More memories of Buccleuch Street. Veterinary Faculty News Issue No 12, February 2001, p7
28. Glasgow Veterinary School 1862-1962 (1962) p6
29. Adair, W, The Glasgow Veterinary College (incorporated) Records of Eighty Years Progress (1941) p11
30. Boden, E, Politics and Practice: The British Veterinary Association, 1882 - 2009 Part 3: 1946 – 1960 p14 http://www.bva.co.uk/public/documents/BVA_History_1945 _1960.pdf (September 2011)
31. Carter, V, ed, Cotchin, E, The Royal Veterinary College London A Bicentenary History, Buckingham (1990) p128

32. Glasgow Veterinary School 1862-1962 (1962) p8
33. Adair, W, The Glasgow Veterinary College (incorporated) Records of Eighty Years Progress (1941) p12
34. Obituary of John Gilruth, The Veterinary Record Vol 49 No 12 (1937) p381
35. The Royal College of Veterinary Surgeons 1844-1944 Centenary Commemoration Number, The Veterinary Record Vol 57 No 51 (1945) pp 599-677 p660
36. Adair, W, The Glasgow Veterinary College (incorporated) Records of Eighty Years Progress (1941) p14
37. Weipers, W, Centenary of the Foundation of the Glasgow Veterinary College. Veterinary Record, (1963) Vol 75 No 3 65-69 p3
38. What are we about in Glasgow for the cure of disease among horses. Southern Press, Friday 5th October (1900) from University of Glasgow Archives Collection DC 144/7/6/1
39. Articles on the Scottish Zoo. Veterinarian, August (1878) from the University of Glasgow Archives Collection DC 144/7/6/1
40. Letter from James Murphy MRCVS Professor of Zoology regarding the closure of Glasgow Zoo, Evening Times, 27th August (1909) University of Glasgow Archives Collection DC 144/7/6/1
41. Adair, W, The Glasgow Veterinary College (incorporated) Records of Eighty Years Progress (1941) p14
42. Glasgow Veterinary School 1862-1962 (1962) p14
43. Agricultural News, Veterinary College Centenary – Celebrations in Glasgow Glasgow Herald 23rd November 1962 University of Glasgow Archives Collection DC 144/7/5/1
44. Obituary of James McCall in the Scottish Farmer 10th November 1915 from the University of Glasgow Archive Collection DC 144/7/1
45. Moss M, Lindsay F, 'We did not feel in any way we were pioneers. the experiences of the first women veterinary students in Glasgow', Newsletter of the University of Glasgow Veterinary Faculty Issue No 10 April 2000 p7
46. Funeral of Principal McCall from The 'Glasgow Herald' 5 Nov 1915
47. The Friends of Glasgow Necropolis http://www.glasgownecropolis.org/ (July 2012)
48. Adair, W, The Glasgow Veterinary College (incorporated) Records of Eighty Years Progress (1941) p14
49. Weipers, W, Half a Century in the Vet Profession (1970s). University of Glasgow Archive Collections ACCN 2051/1/10
50. Adair, W, The Glasgow Veterinary College (incorporated) Records of Eighty Years Progress (1941) p14
51. Glanders www.britannica.com/EBchecked/topic/234796/glanders
52. The Royal College of Veterinary Surgeons 1844-1944 Centenary Commemoration Number, The Veterinary Record Vol 57 No 51 (1945) pp599- 677 p632
53. Adair, W, The Glasgow Veterinary College (incorporated) Records of Eighty Years Progress (1941) p15
54. Adair, W, The Glasgow Veterinary College (incorporated) Records of Eighty Years Progress (1941) pp20-21
55. Transcript of a Video interview of Sir William Weipers with Dr Peter McKenzie, Royal College of Physicians and Surgeons Glasgow Archive Collection RCPSG 18/19 p5
56. Transcript of a Video interview of Sir William Weipers with Dr Peter McKenzie, RCPSG 18/19
57. Glasgow Veterinary School 1862-1962 (1962) p13
58. Adair, W, The Glasgow Veterinary College (incorporated) Records of Eighty Years Progress (1941) p21
59. Carter, V, ed, Cotchin,E, The Royal Veterinary College London A Bicentenary History, Buckingham (1990) p175
60. Marion Stewart http://www.universitystory.gla.ac.uk biography/?id=WH2906&type=P
61. Moss M, Lindsay F, 'We did not feel in any way we were pioneers. The experiences of the first women veterinary students in Glasgow', Newsletter of the University of Glasgow Veterinary Faculty Issue No 10 April 2000 p7

62. Cameron, M. The rise of women in the profession. 2. The 1950s graduate. In Practice. March 2003 pp166-167
63. Glasgow Veterinary School 1862-1962 (1962) p13
64. Adair, W, The Glasgow Veterinary College (incorporated) Records of Eighty Years Progress (1941) p24
65. Wight, J, The Real James Herriot. The Authorised Biography. London (1999) pp74-75
66. Wight, J, The Real James Herriot. The Authorised Biography. London (1999) pp351-352
67. James Alfred Wight http://www.universitystory.gla.ac.uk/biography/?id=WH0090&type =P&o=&start=0&max=20&l= (August 2011)
68. McCreath CP, Obituary Mr EC Straiton, The Veterinary Record Volume 155 Number 20 November 13 (2004) pp644-645
69. Boden E, Eddie Straiton First of the TV vets, The Independent. Wednesday 10th November 2004
70. Glasgow Veterinary School 1862-1962 (1962) p14
71. Carter, V, ed, Cotchin,E, The Royal Veterinary College London A Bicentenary History, Buckingham (1990) p174
72. Glasgow Veterinary School 1862-1962 (1962) p14
73. The history of the RCVS http://www.rcvs.org.uk/about-us/ the-history-of-the-rcvs/(November 2011)
74. Campbell, R, From Buccleuch Street to Barrier Reef, Veterinary Faculty News, Issue 13, September 2001, pp6-7
75. Honorary fellowships for Gardner Murray & Harry Pfaff, Veterinary Faculty News Issue No 17, January 2004 p10
76. Martin, B, Recollections of the Glasgow Veterinary College, The Newsletter of the University of Glasgow Veterinary Faculty, Issue No 18 July 2004, p12
77. Sir William Weipers, the first Dean (1968-1974). The beginning of the Faculty of Veterinary Medicine. Newsletter of the University of Glasgow Veterinary Faculty Issue 25, Summer 2010 p5
78. Armour J, Sir William Weipers: renowned Scots veterinarian Obituary from the Scotsman 19th December 1990
79. Sir William Weipers: renowned Scots veterinarian Silver Jubilee 1949-1974 and the Retiral of the First Director and Dean Sir William Weipers
80. The retirement of William Weipers, College Courant, Martinmas 1974, University of Glasgow Archive Collection DC144/7/5/1
81. Transcript of a Video interview of Sir William Weipers with Dr Peter McKenzie, Royal College of Physicians and Surgeons Glasgow Archive Collection RCPSG 18/19 p35
82. Sir William Weipers, the first Dean (1968-1974). The beginning of the Faculty of Veterinary Medicine. Newsletter of the University of Glasgow Veterinary Faculty Issue 25, Summer 2010 p5
83. Glasgow Veterinary School 1862-1962 (1962) p14
84. Armour J, Sir William Weipers: renowned Scots veterinarian, Obituary from the Scotsman 19th December 1990
85. Transcript of a Video interview of Sir William Weipers with Dr Peter McKenzie, Royal College of Physicians and Surgeons Glasgow Archives Collection RCPSG 18/19 p4
86. Sir William Weipers, the first Dean (1968-1974). The beginning of the Faculty of Veterinary Medicine. Newsletter of the University of Glasgow Veterinary Faculty Issue 25, Summer 2010 p5
87. Weipers, W, Half a century in the Veterinary Profession. Paper given to the Victory Club of the DVA in the mid 70s. University of Glasgow Archives Collection ACCN 2051/1/10
88. Transcript of a Video interview of Sir William Weipers with Dr Peter McKenzie, Royal College of Physicians and Surgeons Glasgow Archives Collection RCPSG 18/19 p55
89. Letter to Sir Hector Hetherington from William Weipers regarding terms for becoming director for the Glasgow Veterinary School, 18th April 1949, from University of Glasgow Archives Collections
90. Brown AL, Moss M, The University of Glasgow :1451-2001 (1996) p87

[91] Douglas, TA, Obituary for John Roberts. The Newsletter of the University of Glasgow Veterinary Faculty Issue 7 April 1998 p3

[92] Wright, N, Betty Blake, University of Glasgow Faculty of Veterinary Medicine Newsletter Issue 24,Winter 2009 p19

[93] Glasgow Veterinary School 1862-1962 (1962) p14

[94] Moss, M, Rankin, M, Richmond L, Who, Where and When: The History & Constitution of the University of Glasgow (2001) p134

[95] Garscube Gazette 30th Edition, January 30 1969

[96] Glasgow Veterinary School 1862-1962 (1962) p3

[97] Garscube Gazette November 1962

[98] Weipers, W, Centenary of the Foundation of the Glasgow Veterinary College Veterinary Record, Vol 75 No. 3 (1963) pp 65-69

[99] 1949 – 1999 Fifty and Forwards Golden Jubilee Celebration (1999)

[100] King, T, Glasgow University Veterinary Practice in Avenue no 10, June 1991 pp 38-39

[101] Bogan JA, Veterinary Medicine, University of Glasgow Newsletter 12th February 1981 pp4-5

[102] Sir William Weipers http://www.universitystory.gla.ac.uk/biography/?id=WH0091&type=P (August 2011)

[103] Jimmy Armour, the sixth Dean (1986-1991) University of Glasgow Faculty of Veterinary Medicine Newsletter Issue 25 Summer 2010 p12

[104] Previous principals of the University of Edinburgh http://www.ed.ac.uk/about/people/officials/previous-principlas (September 2011)

[105] Armour, J, Wright N, Veterinary Medicine in the University of Glasgow (1998) p10

[106] Jimmy Armour, the sixth Dean (1986-1991), University of Glasgow Faculty of Veterinary Medicine Newsletter issue 25 Summer 2010 p12

[107] Gibson N, Victory sealed for the vet school. 'The Evening Times', 1990

[108] Veterinary Education into the 21st Century University of Glasgow Submission in response to The Report of the UGC Working Party under the Chairmanship of Sir Ralph Riley DSc, FRS, 28th March 1989

[109] Armour, J, Wright N, Veterinary Medicine in the University of Glasgow (1998) p11

[110] Carter, V, ed, Cotchin, E, The Royal Veterinary College London A Bicentenary History, Buckingham (1990) p207

[111] Murray, M, From the Boy Pathologist to Professorial Prodigy to Dean: the Retirement of Norman Gray Wright BVMS, PhD, DVM, FIBiol, FRC Path, FRSE, MRCVS. Veterinary Faculty News. The Newsletter of the University of Glasgow Veterinary Faculty, Issue 12, February 2001 p2

[112] Norman Wright, the seventh and longest serving Dean (1991-1999), University of Glasgow Faculty of Veterinary Medicine Newsletter issue 25 Summer 2010 p14

[113] Yam, P, Stricek, A, What happened at Fifty and Forwards. Newsletter of the University of Glasgow Veterinary Faculty Issue No 10 April 2000 pp4-5

[114] A successful year for the Nursing School. University of Glasgow Faculty of Veterinary Medicine Newsletter issue 25 Summer 2010 p21

[115] Rankin, M, Dale, V Overseas Vets at Glasgow Part 1: 1862-1948 Veterinary Faculty News Issue No 20 August 2006 p13

[116] A Brief History World class and proud of our heritage 2009

[117] Yam, P, Glasgow gets AVMA Approval! Newsletter of the University of Glasgow Veterinary Faculty Issue No. 10 April 2000 p2

[118] AVMA approved for another 7 years. Veterinary Faculty News Issue No 21 April 2007 p1

[119] Personal reflections of Mary Stewart University of Glasgow Faculty of Veterinary Medicine Newsletter Issue 25 Summer 2010 p6

[120] Vail, A, Hewitt, A, Record amount raised for charities in GUVMA rodeo. Veterinary Faculty News Issue No 18, July 2004 p1

[121] E-learning and CLIVE http://www.gla.ac.uk/schools/vet/studentstaff/forstudents/e-learningandclive/ (August 2011)

[122] CLIVE http://www.clive.ed.ac.uk/ (August 2011)

[123] E-Learning at Garscube and beyond. University of Glasgow Faculty of Veterinary Medicine Newsletter Issue 23, Spring 2009 p10

[124] 'Objective, Structured, Clinical, Examination': OSCEs are the way forward. University of Glasgow Faculty of Veterinary Medicine Newsletter Issue 24, Winter 2009 p12-13

[125] Public Health in Scotland. Veterinary Faculty Newsletter November 1997 p4

[126] New Masters Degree in Veterinary Public Health to be available from 2006. Veterinary Faculty News Issue No 19 October 2005 p7

[127] Another first for Glasgow … Official Veterinarian Course approved by FSA & MHS. Vet Faculty News Issue No 20 August 2006 p10

[128] The 'virtual abattoir' aids teaching, University of Glasgow Faculty of Veterinary Medicine Newsletter Issue 25 Summer 2010 p23

[129] Veterinary Biosciences Undergraduate Study http://www.gla.ac.uk/media/media_87218_en.pdf (August 2011)

[130] The Veterinary Biosciences degree is underway. An innovative programme and a first for Scotland. Faculty of Veterinary Medicine Newsletter. Issue 23, Spring 2009 p4

[131] Sir James Black, Doctor and pharmacologist, Obituary Sir James Black, Herald Scotland, 23rd March 2010

[132] World Changing Project. "Winning the Nobel Prize for Medicine in 1988 ."In University of Glasgow World Changing,University of Glasgow, 2010. http://www.worldchanging.glasgow.ac.uk/article/?id=6 (accessed September 14, 2011)

[133] Obituary Sir James Black, University of Glasgow Faculty of Veterinary Medicine Issue 25 Summer 2010 p27

[134] Obituary Ian McIntyre, Herald Scotland 29th March 2008 check author

[135] Murray, M et al, WFH Jarett,Obituary for William Jarrett, Veterinary Record 2011;169:474-475

[136] Scientific discoveries through the decades. University of Glasgow Faculty of Veterinary Medicine Newsletter Issue 25 Summer 2010 p13

[137] Historic Moredun Agreement Glasgow-Moredun collaboration on food animal health. Veterinary Faculty News Issue No. 20 August 2006 p2

[138] Moredun Research Institute Joint Research projects http://www.moredun.org.uk/research/scientific-partnerships/university-of-glasgow/joint-research-projects (August 2011)

[139] University of Glasgow RAE 2008 http://www.gla.ac.uk/about/facts/rae/

[140] MMoss, M, Garscube http://www.gla.ac.uk/schools/vet/aboutus/history/garscube/ (August 2011)

[141] Armour, J, Wright N, Veterinary Medicine in the University of Glasgow (1998) p5

[142] Past Secretaries Holders of Office of The Secretary of State for Scotland since 1707 http://www.scotlandoffice.gov.uk/scotlandoffice/63.47.html (August 2011)

[143] Farming News August 1960, p23 University of Glasgow Archive Collection DC144/7/6/1

[144] Personal reflections of Mary Stewart University of Glasgow Faculty of Veterinary Medicine Newsletter Issue 25 Summer 2010 p6

[145] Jimmy Armour, the sixth Dean (1986-1991) University of Glasgow Faculty of Veterinary Medicine Newsletter issue 25 Summer 2010 p12

[146] Glasgow Veterinary School 1862-1962 (1962) p15

[147] Parkins, J, More Land for Cochno, The Newsletter of the Glasgow Veterinary Faculty Issue No 6 1997 pp1-3

[148] Parkins, J, Cochno Farm & Research Centre moves with the times! Veterinary Faculty News Issue No 17, January 2004

[149] Cochno Facilities http://www.gla.ac.uk/faculties/vet/cochno/ (August 2011)

[150] Cochno has a 'face-lift'. University of Glasgow Faculty of Veterinary Medicine Newsletter Issue 24, Winter 2009 p7

[151] Murray, M, Major Building Pro-active Development Fund August 2011

[152] MacMillan, A, Development Fund Builds for the Future. Veterinary Faculty News, Issue No 16 July 2003, pp8-9

[153] Where are they now? … Tim Greet (1976) Veterinary Faculty News. The Newsletter of the University of Glasgow Veterinary Faculty, Issue 12, February 2001 p6

[154] Some people make the same mistake a hundred times and call it experience. University of Glasgow Faculty of Veterinary Medicine Newsletter issue 25 Summer 2010 p8

[155] Honorary Professorship for Tim Greet (1976) Veterinary Faculty News Issue No 18, July 2004 p14

[156] Macmillan, A, Reunion News "Glancing Back, Looking Forwards" Invitation to a homecoming party for all alumni. Veterinary Faculty News Issue No 18, July 2004 p10

[157] Yam, P, Alumni Celebratory Weekend – Glancing Back Looking Forward! Veterinary Faculty News Issue No. 19 October 2005 p9

[158] A new £10m hospital by 2008! Veterinary Faculty News Issue No. 19 October 2005 p1

[159] VArchitects appointed to design new 'green' hospital. Vet School Campaign Newsletter Issue No 1 December 2005 p3

[160] Archial's Small Animal Hospital Wins Civic Trust Award www.glasgowarchitecture.co.uk/small_animal_hospital.htm (August 2011)

[161] Doggie Dawdle Vet School Campaign Newsletter Issue No 2 July 2006

[162] Scottish Parliament welcomes opening of new Small Animal Hospital at the University of Glasgow. University of Glasgow Faculty of Veterinary Medicine Newsletter Issue 24, Winter 2009 pp2-3

[163] Small Animal Hospital Officially Open University of Glasgow Faculty of Veterinary Medicine Newsletter issue 25 Summer 2010 p28

[164] Archial's Small Animal Hospital Wins Civic Trust Award www.glasgowarchitecture.co.uk/small_animal_hospital.htm (August 2011)

[165] A flagship for clinical provision - Glasgow unveils its new small animal hospital. Veterinary Record 2009 165:333

[166] The future growth of the Vet School with particular reference to the expected pressure on the University in 1965 and after. University of Glasgow Archives Collection ACCN 2773/12/1-2

[167] RCVS Visitation: general information requested in Paper 1 and Paper 2 University of Glasgow Archives Collection ACCN 2773/12/3

[168] Veterinary Faculty News The Newsletter of the University of Glasgow Veterinary Faculty, Issue No 13, September 2001 6,780,000,for New Research Centre for the Institute of Comparative Medicine p1

[169] Henry Wellcome Institute for Comparative Medicine CP98/293 http://www.gla.ac.uk/services/estates/projectdirectory/completedprojects/henrywellcomeinstituteforcomparativemedicine/ (May 2012)

[170] Wight, J, The Real James Herriot. The Authorised Biography. Penguin Books London (1999) p355

[171] Glasgow Veterinary School 1862-1962 (1962) p16

[172] Letter from William Weipers to Dr Hutcheson, Secretary of Court, University of Glasgow, 20th November 1962 University of Glasgow Archives Collection ACCN 2773/14/1

[173] Building Developments. University of Glasgow Faculty of Veterinary Medicine Newsletter issue 25 Summer 2010 p14

[174] Dawda K Jawara http://universitystory.gla.ac.uk/biography/?id=WH5233&type=P&o=&start=0&max=20&d= (August 2011)

[175] Campbell, B 'A Lion for the Emperor' Veterinary Faculty News Issue No 20 August 2006 p13

[176] Links with Africa continue. University of Glasgow Faculty of Veterinary Medicine Newsletter issue 25 Summer 2010 p16

Glasgow Vets 1862–2012

150

Celebrating 150 years of veterinary excellence